CW01213673

It's not the Trauma, It's the Drama

Stories by a
Chicago Fire Department Paramedic

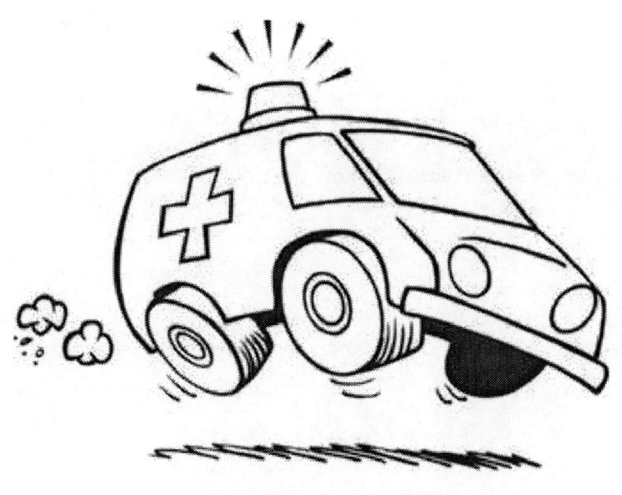

MARJORIE LEIGH BOMBEN

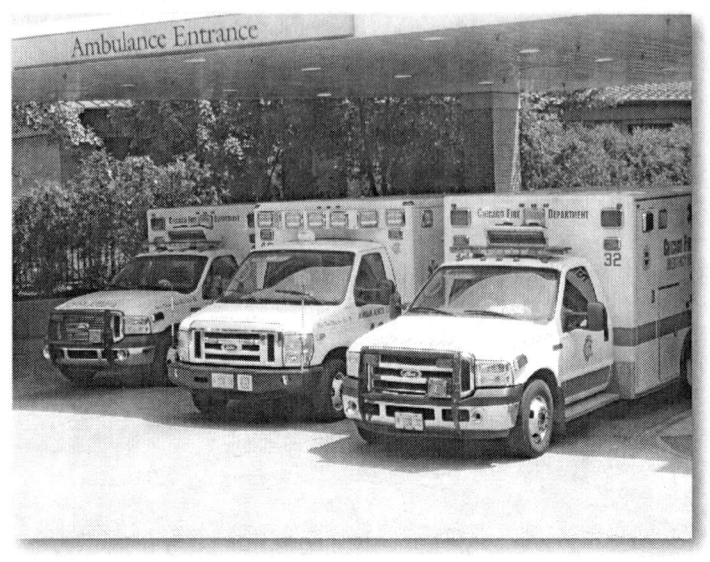

Text © 2015 by Marjorie Leigh Bomben
Photos © 2015 by Marjorie Leigh Bomben except cover photo, author photo and photo on page 41 courtesy of Ruth G. Sikes. Candidate photo on page 5 courtesy of Bob Silverman. Courtesy of Engine 109's quarters, photo on page 60 of the old quarters of Engine 109. The staircase photo on page 61 courtesy of firefighter/EMT Rich Papez.

All rights reserved. No part of this book may be reproduced in any form or by any means, electronic or mechanical, including photocopying, recording or by any information storage and retrieval system, without permission from the author.

Inquiries should be sent to:
mbomben@yahoo.com

Library of Congress Cataloging-in-Publication Data
Bomben, Marjorie Leigh

ISBN-13: 9781500741785
ISBN-10: 1500741787
Library of Congress Control Number: 2015901031
CreateSpace Independent Publishing Platform
North Charleston, South Carolina
Printed in the United States of America

This book is dedicated to the paramedics
of the Chicago Fire Department

Acknowledgements

I am grateful for my Mother's indispensable advice, her editing and encouragement.

A special thanks to Rosemary Burke for granting me permission to share "Don's Story."

Contents

Introduction · ix
My First Trauma · 1
Down From the Unknown Cause · 6
Just Another Day at the Office · 13
You Have to Pay for That · 16
I've Been Shot · 20
Communicating with the Spirits · 24
The Wrench · 32
Don's Story · 35
Badge of Honor · 42
La Tortuga · 46
The Old Quarters of Ambulance 34 · 55
Truck Guys · 62
You've Got My Eye · 69
Only a Cut, Please · 75
Naked Man · 78
Oh, Shit · 84
A Heck of a Party · 87
Imagine · 90
The Specter · 94
Thinking Outside of the Box · 101
The Democratic Committeemen · 107

"I guarantee I've had a weirder day than you."

Introduction

CHICAGO HAS ONE of the highest murder rates and some of the busiest ambulances in the United States. Chicago Fire Department ambulances respond to over 300,000 calls per year. Paramedics can and often do work their entire twenty-four-hour shift without any sleep, operating in some of the most dangerous neighborhoods in the country. Gain an insider's view into what it's really like to work on a Chicago Fire Department (CFD) ambulance.

Paramedics tell stories, whether they're socializing off duty or hanging out at the hospital after a call. What happened on the last run leads to a crazy story about what occurred during the last shift.

When the old-timers, coworkers of mine who had been on the job for over thirty years, began to retire, they took their treasure trove of stories and experiences with them. What a loss!

It is for this reason that I put pen to paper. Some of the stories are comical; some not for the weak of heart. All of them are true; however, some names, locations and details have been changed.

After over thirty years of working for the CFD, I have forgotten much more than I have retained. *It's Not the Trauma, It's the Drama* documents some of the stories that have stuck with me and that I feel compelled to share.

My First Trauma

It was 1983. I had been living in Chicago for a few years and was fresh out of paramedic school when I was hired by the Chicago Fire Department. I came to the department a clean slate, a naive kid from the suburbs. Nothing from my paramedic books had prepared me for what I would encounter working on a Chicago Fire Department ambulance.

I was called a candidate paramedic for one year, evaluated by my peers, then hopefully would earn fire paramedic status. Crisp uniform with razor sharp creases still in the pants and that look of someone who is lost but is afraid to ask for directions was a dead give away of my candidate status.

Working on the job for over a month had not produced anything resembling a real emergency; the fact was, we got a tremendous amount of calls for non-life threatening issues. Thankfully the learning curve was steep due to the high volume of runs we went on. Before getting my first real emergency, I was able to gain some experience. The ambulance gods must have been watching over me.

How sorry I felt for my fellow candidates who had some horrendous call on their first day. The kindly pat on the shoulder from their partner who was giving them that knowing look…"Kid, some day you'll get the hang of it," and the deer in the head lights expression on their face.

My first real trauma occurred while working on Ambulance 33. My partner Stan, a paramedic officer on duty and plumber off duty, lovingly referred to his rig, Ambulance 33, as "tirty tree, pair o' trees."

It was dark, about three in the morning on a warm, humid July night on the West Side of Chicago. Two cars had been drag racing down Ogden Boulevard. One car contained several men, the other their female counterparts plus two young children. The latter was the car that had hit a light pole at a high rate of speed.

Making our way south on Ogden toward Kedzie Avenue, I could see multi-colored lights pulsating in a sea of darkness. Two ambulances were already on the scene treating the children. The car looked like it had just come out of a trash compactor.

As we approached with our stretcher in tow, my field of vision was limited to the car from which firefighters were extricating a woman. It seemed as if a flashlight were casting a beam of light through the darkness onto the vehicle. I had no awareness of anything outside this circle of light. It was the strangest sensation. I didn't know I had tunnel vision, I thought. This cannot be good. Am I panicking?

I didn't have much time to ponder my mental state as we were handed a backboard with what appeared to be a body on it. After placing the board on our awaiting stretcher, we headed for the ambulance as the firefighters checked the wreckage for more victims. "There's another one in here," one of the firefighters said.

"We can take two," Stan replied as they removed a crumpled figure from under the dashboard. How was it possible for a person to come out of that small area?

Out she did come.

After loading our first patient into the rig, the firefighters placed the second victim on a backboard and positioned her on the bench seat in the back of the ambulance.

Surveying this ghastly lineup, I saw that the woman on the stretcher was breathing. It looked as if her body were on backward. Her right eyeball was delicately laying on her cheek, hanging by a thread—a perfect glistening globe. The woman on the bench seat was also breathing, her limbs were at unnatural angles. She had two open fractures in each extremity. Not only was the bone broken, but it was also protruding from an open wound caused by the bone puncturing the skin, hence the name "open fracture." Thankfully for them, both women were unconscious.

I didn't know where to start. I would never have imagined that bodies could be in that condition and still be alive. This scenario was not in the books. Vital signs, bandaging, oxygen, IV's, heart monitor… as soon as I began, everything fell into place. Then it was off to the hospital. It all seemed so futile. They could not possibly survive, as ultimately they did not, but it was not my decision who to treat or not to treat. I did my job as best as I could.

Stan got behind the wheel. This was a major concern, as he drove like a maniac when we were just going to get fuel. I was in a constant state of terror while working with him. There we were on the West Side of Chicago, the murder capital of the city, and I was more afraid of Stan's driving than of the neighborhood.

Stan's beloved ambulance "tirty tree" had a lot of character. In other words, it was falling apart. There was a hole in the floor of the patient compartment the size of a dinner platter, the street visible, whizzing by below, and a sister hole in the floor of the front passenger seat. It did, however, provide some fresh air, as the air conditioning didn't work. The side mirrors and front fender were held on using white medical tape. The two-inch tape was the go-to quick fix for anything that broke on the ambulance, from cinching closed the glove compartment to holding together vital parts of the rig.

The patient compartment, or "box" was attached to the front of the ambulance by what appeared to be a couple of flimsy wires that I was sure were going to snap at any moment. The back of the ambulance had a life of its own, careening back and forth and up and down out of sync with the front, which confidently surged forward toward Mount Sinai Hospital. I called the hospital en route on our telemetry radio to alert them that we were bringing in two severe trauma patients.

Of the utmost importance is a smooth delivery of your report to the hospital; painting a picture of the scene and describing patient injuries, condition and treatment in a precise, yet brief manner. We were taught this technique in paramedic school, but once the radio is in your hand, all sorts of disasters were likely to occur—giving information out of order, mispronouncing words, neglecting to mention pertinent information, or repeating information already delivered. The worst of all is the "freeze" during which a long awkward bout of silence occurs because you are actually having some sort of brain seizure along with sweating and heart palpitations brought on by a complete loss of knowing where you are in your radio report.

Telling the novel version of the story instead of the Cliff Notes version is also a big mistake. I have witnessed many a telemetry nurse roll her eyes, put down the phone, and perform several procedures on patients before returning to the telemetry console and finish listening to the transmission. Once you have earned a reputation of giving a good radio report, respect by the doctors and nurses at the hospitals can be at hand.

After the hospital has been alerted that a trauma patient is on the way, the trauma surgeon is paged. The trauma doc is a beast to be reckoned with. Often a bit arrogant, he looks down on the lowly uneducated paramedic—more of a stooge than a fellow medical professional, which can be proven by a disastrous telemetry report booming throughout the emergency department.

I called the hospital en route. For the first time, I felt secure in the delivery of my radio report. It was as if a divine hand had been upon my shoulder, as something I could not describe possessed me—it was perfect and effortless. The tone of the voice on the other end of the radio seemed to doubt me when I gave an account of the injuries sustained.

A team of doctors, nurses, residents and medical students had assembled in the trauma room awaiting our arrival. We transferred our patients onto hospital gurneys. The trauma surgeon slowly circled one of the beds, lifting a limb here and a limb there. The sweetest words I have ever heard floated out of his lips. "I will never doubt the paramedics again."

IT'S NOT THE TRAUMA, IT'S THE DRAMA

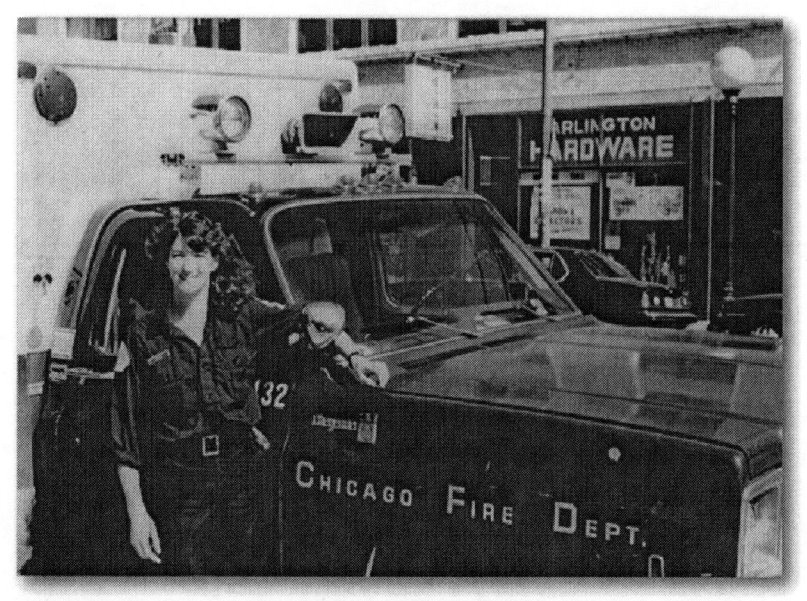

Candidate paramedic, 1983

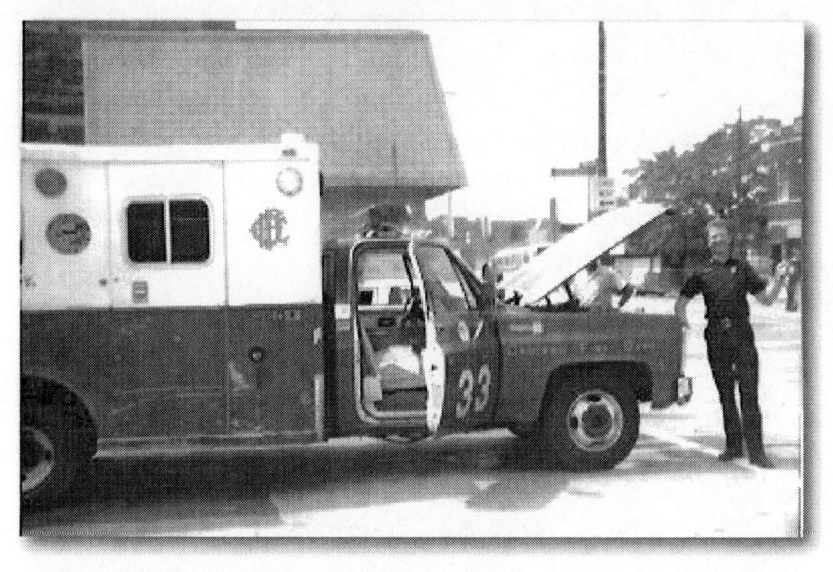

The old Ambulance 33 after an engine fire was extinguished, 1984

Down From the Unknown Cause

I SHOULD HAVE BEEN scared. However, I found the man who was crawling through the passenger side window toward me an annoyance, like a fly you swat away that keeps returning and buzzing about your head. My only thought was to rid myself of this intrusive pest.

The year was 1985. It was about five in the morning on a stiflingly hot August morning. The heat and humidity had the effect of making me feel like a Petri dish, ripe for growing some moldy culture. Smells emanating from my patients adhered to me, finding a hold in the salty moisture on my body. Stale alcohol breath, the fetid smell of putrid feet and the coppery aroma of blood clung to me. I couldn't wait to get home and scrub my body, hoping to remove several layers of skin to feel clean again.

I was working on Ambulance 10, which is located on the West Side at Pulaski and West End Avenue. Barry and I had gotten a call for a six month old with difficulty breathing.

"Did you take her temperature?"

"No."

"Why not?"

"I don't have a thermometer, I can't afford it." Noticing the track marks on mom's arms, she clearly could afford her drug of choice. After a thorough examination, the baby clearly had nothing more than a cold.

"Do you want to go to the hospital?"

"Yeah." We loaded up mom and the baby. I was driving with Barry in the back as we made our way toward Mount Sinai Hospital.

IT'S NOT THE TRAUMA, IT'S THE DRAMA

It was so ridiculous, calling 911 for a baby with a cold. I decided to take a stand, as small and inconsequential as it was, I was not going to turn on the lights and siren.

I knew it would not make any difference—people would still call for non-emergencies—but it somehow made me feel a little better. There was no traffic at that hour anyway. I momentarily slowed at a red light at Lake and Pulaski. I checked both ways; the intersection was clear. I began to proceed through, mulling over the lost precious thirty minutes of sleep I would not be getting, when out of nowhere a man appeared in front of the ambulance frantically waving his arms.

As I came to a stop, he ran to the passenger side window, which was open because we had no air conditioning.

"Some guy fell out," he said. "Fell out" is a West Side term for passed out.

"Where is he?" I asked.

Pointing in the direction of the man down, he said, "Right around the corner in the street."

"Ambulance 10 to dispatch."

"10 go."

"There is a report of a man down at Lake and Pulaski on the southeast corner. Can you send another ambulance?"

"Ambulance 15, take the man down from the unknown cause on the southeast corner of Lake and Pulaski."

As I began to speak, to tell him another ambulance was on the way, he proceeded to open the passenger side door. Instinctively, I gunned the ambulance with the guy still clinging to the outside of the door, then I slammed on the brakes, hoping the force would knock him off; however he held tight. I tried this a couple of times. The door would start to close when I floored it, and it would spring open when I slammed on the brakes. I alternated between stepping on the gas and slamming on the brakes, the door flapping like a berserk bird. On the third try, the door snapped shut and he began to climb through the open window toward me.

"Hey, get out of here!" Barry, alerted by my erratic driving had stuck his head through the small square opening that connected the front and back of the ambulance to see what was going on. It had the immediate effect of my friend running off, as I assumed he had thought I was alone. Ambulance 15 never found anyone down from any cause, known or unknown, at that location.

• • •

My next workday, I was on Ambulance 33, which is housed in Engine 107's quarters, at 13th Street and California Avenue. I was working with Dave Milner. Dave was short and fair, with tiny almond-shaped eyes set above an upturned nose. A wisp of blond hair flew about his balding head.

"Ambulance 33, take the man down from the unknown cause outside the bar at 2345 South California."

We rolled up to find our victim laying face down on the sidewalk, seemingly unresponsive. "Hey, buddy, wake up, are you OK?" I said as I shook him with no response. We saw no signs of trauma and gently rolled him onto his back. The stale smell of alcohol assaulted my nose; this guy was wasted. We grabbed the stretcher and hefted him onto the gurney.

Once in the ambulance, I checked his vital signs and blood sugar. They were within normal limits. I lit it up and headed over to Saint Anthony Hospital. En route, I happened to glance in the rearview mirror.

"Oh my G-d!" Dave was in an epic battle in the back of the rig with the patient who had suddenly awakened. Veering to the curb, I slammed it into "park" and then ran to the back of the rig. I flung open both back doors. I assumed that the patient had been confused when he woke up and just wanted out of the rig, I was hoping he would see the doors were open and make his escape. I yelled at him to get out, however, he wouldn't budge. They had ahold of each other, and I wasn't sure who had whom. I jumped into the back of the ambulance and began to pry the patient's hands off of Dave. Suddenly our ward let go, stood up to his full height and took a mighty swing at me. I turned my head just in time, but still received a glancing blow on the side of my face. He then disappeared out of the back of the rig.

"Are you OK?" I asked Dave.

"Yeah, how about you?"

"I turned my head just in time to not get cracked full in the face. How does it look?"

"A little swollen, I'm going to call for the police and a field chief." We headed over to Mount Sinai Emergency Department to make out a police report; Dave thought I should get my face looked at. My field chief asked me if I wanted to be seen at the hospital. I said I thought I would be fine. My cheek was only slightly red and a bit swollen; it was really no big deal. After completing the reports, I went back to work.

That next week I was working on Ambulance 33 again with Dave. Dave and I were not a good combination. Like a marriage, in my opinion, sometimes opposites work best, one filling in where the other is lacking. "Good cop, bad cop" sounds cliché but it works quite well. When one paramedic is crabby, the other makes up for it by killing them with kindness. We, however, did not have this dynamic; we were both really crabby.

I had been on the department for five years. At this five year milestone the novelty of the job had worn off, and reality began seeping in. People call for BS.

It's not out of the ordinary to work a whole twenty-four-hour shift, generally over twenty calls, and then find that not one of them actually needed an ambulance. At that point in my career, I had neither the maturity nor the will to accept the inevitability of the situation. You can never win by losing your cool. People will always call again and again for the same baloney. It makes absolutely no difference if you are rude to them; they will still want to go to the hospital, and will probably call back the next day for the same silliness. The only effect of being nasty is that you become angry and agitated, which could lead to a complaint from the patient and possibly a suspension.

The fact of the matter is that we are social services on wheels, occasionally interrupted by an actual emergency. I needed to find some way to come to terms with this, or find another vocation. I was going to school part time—I had decided that I couldn't do this for much longer. I was so angry that either I was going to kill someone, or someone was going to kill me.

"Ambulance 33, take the person down from the unknown cause at 1411 South Albany, floor three." Dave and I hiked up the three flights of stairs and knocked on the door. The patient's mother, a middle-aged woman, answered.

"We had an argument and my son 'fell out'," she stated. Our twenty-three year old patient sat on the couch with his eyes closed. He had no pertinent medical history.

"Hey mister, what's the matter?" I said as I gently shook his shoulder. There was no response. Dave checked his vital signs and blood sugar, they were within normal limits. I gently ran my finger across his eyelashes to check his corneal reflex. If his eyelid twitched, he was awake; if it did not, he was actually unconscious. His eyelid twitched, so we knew he was feigning unconsciousness.

Dave loudly stated that this was a bunch of crap. I really didn't want to carry this guy down three flights of stairs because he was upset over an argument with his mother. I told him that I knew he was awake, that he was wasting our time, as there were sick people we could have been tending to. He needed to open his eyes and get up. Well, he did just that.

Bolting up from the couch, he proceeded to chase us down the stairs, threatening to kill us. Once outside, we vaulted into the rig and locked the doors. We were going to make it! However, Dave began to fumble with the key—he couldn't get it in the ignition.

"He's coming," I relayed to Dave. The guy was at my side of the rig. He tried the door. Finding it locked, he picked up a brick.

"He has a brick, come on." The rig coughed to life, I ducked as Dave peeled out, my window shattered and glass flew everywhere.

Dave told dispatch that we were out of service due to an "accident" and needed our field chief and the police to meet us at Mount Sinai Hospital because I had caught some shards of glass in my neck.

Thankfully, my injuries were superficial. I checked into the emergency department anyway, this time informing my field chief that I was laying up. I had been on the job for over five years and had never had anything like that happen. In a two-week period, I experienced two assaults and one attempted assault. I just wanted to get my doctor's note and go home. I had had enough.

• • •

Chicago Fire Department paramedics work in some of the most dangerous neighborhoods in the country. At all hours of the day and night, it's just the two of us. We have no weapons—nothing to defend ourselves with. Sure, we are street-smart and take precautions. For instance, always say, "hey, how's it going," to anyone and everyone as you make your way from the ambulance to the patient. If someone is giving you a hard time on a run, ask him to help you do something, such as holding the stretcher or keep gapers at bay. And never stand in front of a door while you are knocking on it, someone may shoot through it.

A dark and grim reality began to seep into my consciousness. No matter how careful I was, if someone wanted to get me, what's to stop them? I was a sitting duck. I had never looked at my job that way before, and it scared me. I don't do scared.

Contributing to the problem was my poor attitude and bedside manner. I have since grown up a bit and learned to be kind. A show of concern, no matter how ridiculous the complaint is, has the desired effect—the patient will cooperate with you. Everyone will be happy, and you can move on, all in one piece. No matter what, we should not have to worry about our safety, but it is the sad reality of the job. Today, paramedics are attacked on an almost daily basis. It has recently become a felony to assault a paramedic.

I took my time returning to duty. After a couple of weeks off, I was back on Ambulance 33. My neck was fine, but my mental state was not. I had purchased some pepper spray. Feeling the weight of it in my pocket gave me some much-needed confidence and peace of mind.

On my first day back I was presented with a gift from the firefighters, all wrapped up with a bow. It was a Styrofoam brick. "Thanks guys, very thoughtful!" I said. I told them that I had bought some pepper spray. The response was, "will it stop bricks?" So much for my peace of mind.

Just Another Day at the Office

I WAS ON "TIRTY tree, pair o' trees" again, working with my partner/plumber friend, Stan. Stan was a nice enough guy, but he didn't have a great sense of humor. I would expect that being assigned to Ambulance 33 and getting hammered for twenty-four hours and then going to his side job rodding out sewage pipes could tend to make one crabby, but certainly not squeamish.

The fire in the second-floor apartment of the three-story brick building was almost out. Stan and I had been dozing in the rig, standing by at the fire, yet ready to snap into action if the occasion should occur. So far it had not occurred.

Two firefighters approached the rig. They were sweating, covered in soot from head to toe, and breathing heavily. They looked dreadfully pale. Each was holding the end of a black body bag that hung heavily between them as they made their way toward the ambulance. I opened the back doors, and they placed the bag on the stretcher.

"What have you got there?" Stan inquired.

"We found two kids—crispy critters. They're small, so we put them both in one bag.

We were overhauling when Ed stepped on something hard. He heard a crack. It was the head of one of the kids. That's how we were able to find them."

"There was so much debris that I couldn't see anything. I didn't mean to step on him," Ed insisted. Ed did not look well.

"Are you OK?" I asked.

"Yeah, yeah, fine." The poor guy did not look fine. He looked like he was going to pass out. "It's not your fault," I said. With that, the guys disappeared.

Stan and I transported the kids over to Saint Anthony Hospital to be pronounced. We wheeled the stretcher with the body bag on it into a room. I pulled the curtain closed as Stan began to unzip the bag.

"I can't do it."

Baffled, I asked, "Can't do what?"

"I can't take them out."

I am ashamed to say this now, but I actually found this to be amusing. Stan had five years of seniority on me, amounting to several more years of seeing horrendous things, plus all that raw sewage. What was his problem?

"Oh, for G-d's sake, I got it." I said.

Stan immediately vanished from the room, pulling the curtain closed behind him.

I unzipped the bag; the kids had been laid head to toe. One was maybe three years old and the other was about five. No telling what sex they were if you know anything about crispy critters. Critters of the crispy kind are burnt beyond recognition. They are way overcooked, charred black and stiff as a board. With gloved hands, I picked the smaller one up and laid him on the hospital gurney. I went for the second one, but when I lifted him up the top of his head fell off, spilling cooked brains that resembled gray scrambled eggs into the body bag. "Shit."

Back at the firehouse I had a nasty mess to clean up, and I was not happy about it.

I had the hose out on the apparatus floor and was spraying brains out of the body bag, watching them float down a little river of water, spin, and then go down the drain. It struck me then, that I was spraying a kid's brain down a drain and I didn't even care. What was wrong with me? Was I some kind of a monster? I tried to picture the kid riding a bike, perhaps, or playing at the playground. Still nothing. Either this was the perfect job for me, or there was something really wrong with me. Maybe it was both.

• • •

To function, paramedics must be able to emotionally separate themselves from their patients. This can either come naturally or can be learned through experience. In the face of mayhem, how unhelpful it is to be as upset or as panicked as the patient.

Some people might perceive this as being cold or heartless, but in our line of work, it's a necessity. However, it is not an exact science. It's particularly difficult when a patient—especially a child—reminds us of a loved one. Paramedics rarely let this curtain between their personal and professional lives fall.

Twenty years later, I was on Ambulance 46, wheeling a patient into the emergency department at Swedish Covenant Hospital. Several CFD ambulances were lined up in the hospital bay. As we rolled through door, a paramedic walked out, I spun my head around in confusion.

"Stan?" I asked. I knew it couldn't be, as he had retired the year before. This guy looked exactly the same as Stan had twenty years ago.

"No, Ryan," he replied. He was Stan's son. Ryan must have been around the same age as those burnt kids were some twenty years earlier. That is why Stan couldn't touch them.

For me, dealing with pediatric cases was no different then dealing with adults; the patients were just smaller. I did what had to be done and moved on without any emotional turmoil. At that time, I had no children; it had just been another day at the office.

You Have to Pay for That

It was a hot summer day in the predominately Mexican neighborhood of Little Village. The smell of tortilla chips was thick in the air; it emanated from a nearby factory. Kids rode their bikes on crowded sidewalks. Residents pulled out lawn chairs to sit in front of their apartments in an attempt to catch a fleeting breeze and *observer a la gente*, (i.e., people watch). The year was 1986. I was working on Ambulance 34 with Brian Cheevers who was known to the neighborhood kids as "Otro Bruce," English translation, "Other Bruce." The actual Bruce, Bruce Parker, worked on the previous shift. Apparently, to the kids, all the paramedics were some form of a Bruce. Hence I was working with Otro Bruce for my twenty-four-hour shift. The day started off unusually quiet with no runs for several hours. That might seem like a good thing, but if you had been on the department for any length of time, you would know without a doubt, not only is this not good, you would know that somehow you would have to pay for those few precious hours of peace and quiet.

"Brian, you have a front phone," the overhead blared. Brian/Otro Bruce picked up the phone.

"We have to go for PMs," (preventive maintenance for the ambulance, an oil change, etc.) Brian called dispatch to let them know we were out of service and heading over to the shops. We hopped in the rig and made our way toward 31st and Sacramento.

We had driven about a mile and a half when we came upon a three-story brick building on fire; it appeared to be abandoned with most of the windows boarded up. The building was fully involved. It was unusual that someone hadn't already called 911. However, it was early in the morning and many people would still be sleeping. Brian immediately informed dispatch. Fire companies were on the way.

There used to be a lot of abandoned buildings in the Little Village neighborhood. Many mysteriously ended up engulfed in flames, probably for insurance purposes. The Office of Fire Investigation guys used to say that the official cause of those fires was rats with matches.

Brian told dispatch that we would remain on the scene for the time being and then head on over to the shops after the fire was out. It was routine for an ambulance to be assigned to a fire because one might be needed for an injured firefighter or civilian fire victims. This seemed like a pretty straightforward abandoned/unoccupied building fire. "We'll be on our way to the shops shortly," Brian said as he put his head back and closed his eyes. Sirens wailed, hoses were led out, and the firefighters went to work.

There seemed to be a never-ending procession of firefighters delivering to us their precious load. A family, most of them children, had occupied what had appeared to be an abandoned building.

Little limp and unconscious bodies, all in severe respiratory distress or cardiac arrest were lined up on the bench seat, the stretcher, any place we could fit them. Brian had called for more ambulances for what seemed like hours ago. None had arrived. We were simultaneously doing CPR, ventilating and administering oxygen to six children, all of whom appeared to be under the age of five. We didn't have enough equipment or hands. We were able to commandeer one firefighter to help us.

"Ambulance 34 to dispatch."

"Ambulance 34, go."

"Didn't you get my message?" Brian relayed in desperation.

"No, 34, we didn't."

"We need six more ambulances for pediatric fire victims. It would be very helpful if they could get here as soon as possible."

One by one, the ambulances finally arrived. We handed out our patients. It was slow going, as Chicago Fire Department ambulances were few and far between. We still had four victims left but had begun to make some headway with our advanced life-support treatment as we waited for the rest of the ambulances to arrive.

I had just finished intubating a child who was in severe respiratory distress when a police officer appeared at the back of the rig holding an infant. My first thought was, thank G-d she's dead. That's a terrible thing to think, but the baby was completely charred from flames. Burns are terribly painful to endure. It would have been impossible to survive burns of that severity—then the baby cried. Horrified, I pleaded, "Can you please put her in your car and take her to Mount Sinai?"

The hospital was not far, and it seemed like the most expedient way to get the baby the medical attention she needed. We were still overwhelmed with patients and did not have another ambulance on the scene available to transport at that moment. The officer didn't question me and abruptly disappeared with the infant, cradling her in his arms.

As I handed out the last child to Ambulance 10, three firefighters appeared, carrying the limp body of a woman. They laid her down on the ground at the back of our ambulance and began CPR. I jumped out of the back of the rig, IV bag and ET tube in hand and went to work.

"Mike, do you have a cigarette?" I asked.

"You don't smoke."

"I do now."

We were at Cook County Burn Center where we had deposited our last patient. She was the mother of three of the children and the aunt of the other four. Mike was from Ambulance 10, one of the rigs that had come to our assistance. I told him the story of our slow morning with no runs and how we had only made it halfway to PMs. "Hey, you knew you were going to have to pay for that."

IT'S NOT THE TRAUMA, IT'S THE DRAMA

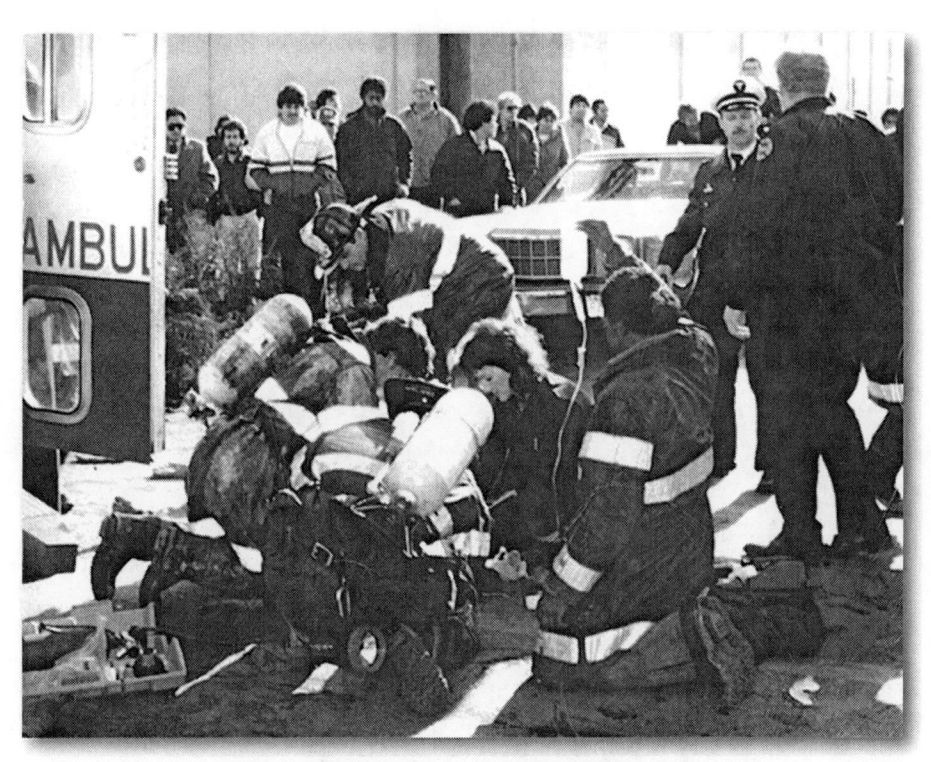

Working on our last patient

I've Been Shot

A CALL AT FIVE in the morning signifies two things—number one, your mind and body are being tortured. You should be in the deepest part of your sleep cycle, REM sleep; vivid dreams, body paralyzed in blissful renewal which is essential for the optimal functioning of all living creatures. And number two, your shift is shot. There is zero possibility of getting any sleep at this point. So face it—even if you had gotten any rest prior to that, you'll never recover from being awakened at that hour. Your body will protest for the rest of the day with a heavy woozy feeling that never abates, like a spoiled child that won't stop whining. Occasionally, very occasionally, for the surprise factor alone, it's worth the rude awakening.

"Ambulance 15, take the shooting at Iowa and Pine." I don't know what it is about Pine Street, but I have had more calls on Pine than on any other street in Chicago. If Pine Street were to magically disappear, my guess is that our run volume would have decreased by a hundred runs per month. We didn't turn on the lights and siren, as we slowly made our way west on Chicago Avenue, sneaking up on the call.

One of the first things we learn in paramedic school is the importance of scene safety. We are taught to never enter a dangerous scene until the police have secured it.

We can't help anyone if we are dead or injured. Blazing in with lights and siren could be a safety hazard as the perpetrator could still be on the scene. If the police had not arrived before us, we would pull over some

IT'S NOT THE TRAUMA, IT'S THE DRAMA

distance away and inform dispatch that we were waiting for the CPD. Thankfully, reassuring blue-and-white lights were visible in the distance.

As we exited the rig, happy chirping birds awaiting an early spring sunrise greeted us. They were blissfully ignorant of the poverty and violence of the neighborhood in which they chose to reside. We made for a cracked sidewalk that was littered with garbage. Two police officers on either side of an elderly African American male guided him toward us.

"We got a call for shots fired. This guy says he's been hit, but we don't see anything." I opened the back of the rig, the officers helped our patient up and we sat him on the bench seat.

"I've been shot, I've been shot I tell you!" he excitedly insisted.

"Where?" I asked.

"I've been shot in the head."

With a gloved hand, I searched our patient's head. I found nothing—not even a scratch.

"Well sir, I don't see anything at all."

"I've been shot! I've been shot in the head I'm telling you!"

"If you'd been shot in the head, you'd be dead."

"Well, I can't die," he firmly stated.

Once you have opened the Pandora's box of talking to patients about any subject other than the exact complaint at hand, you're asking for trouble. You really don't want to get into people's personal lives and thoughts. I have gone this route, and it isn't pretty. But this little old guy was just so cute.

"OK, so why can't you die?" I asked. He looked intently into my eyes and his voice became calm, sweet, and serene as he began to speak.

"Because I's on a mission to save all the peoples of the world—rich and po, black and white. But that nigga who shot me, I'm gonna kill that mothafucker!"

• • •

"Ambulance 15, take the man shot at Augusta and Laramie." It was my next workday at two o'clock in the afternoon, a little early in the day for a shooting, even on the West Side. The police were escorting an adult male toward us as we pulled up. He didn't seem to be in any distress and was walking easily under his own power with no obvious wounds.

"What's your name, buddy?"

"Jerome."

"What happened to ya?" I inquired as we positioned him on the bench seat.

"I heard about five shots. I don't know if I've been hit."

You'd be surprised by the number of people who had no idea whether or not they'd been shot. We would strip off the victim's shirt and pants sometimes finding multiple gunshot wounds that he had no idea he had sustained—or sometimes we would find nothing at all.

I did a visual of our man's head. There wasn't anything obvious. I was about to move on and lift up his shirt when I noticed a trickle of blood coming from behind his left ear. Pulling Jerome's ear forward, I found a small caliber entrance wound. I was dumb-founded. It was not a graze wound. The bullet had entered his skull, but where was it?

Jerome was conscious and alert, answering all questions in an appropriate manner, as if nothing were amiss. After spying the wound, my partner and I gave each other "the look." This was bad. Jerome needed the full treatment. We applied a cervical collar and laid him on a backboard on the stretcher. Vital signs, oxygen, EKG, IV. This guy was going to need a trauma bypass.

A trauma bypass is utilized when a patient's injuries fit a criteria consistent with major trauma that might require a surgeon. The closest hospitals may be bypassed in order to deliver the patient to an accredited trauma center staffed with a trauma team.

Our closest trauma center was Loyola Medical Center which is located in the suburb of Maywood; it was going to be a haul. We contacted Loyola via telemetry radio and relayed a report of our patient's condition, which amazingly, was just fine.

As we made our way to the trauma center, I expected him to crash at any moment. I rechecked his vital signs. My eyes were glued to the heart monitor as I tried to keep a conversation going in order to assess his level of consciousness. However, all Jerome wanted to talk about was his nose.

"My nose is stuffed up. Can I blow my nose?" he asked. Picturing him blowing his brains out through his nose, it was out of the question, as I had no idea where the bullet was.

"Can I blow my nose, man? I need to blow."

"No, you absolutely can't blow your nose."

"Man, just give me a Kleenex."

"No, Jerome, you can't blow. There's a bullet somewhere in your head."

"I'm fine, let me blow my nose." This went on all the way to the hospital. It was getting really annoying.

"Hey, can you step on it?" I asked my partner.

We delivered Jerome to the ED, and transferred him onto a hospital gurney. X-rays were first up. I was definitely hanging around for the results. The trauma surgeon slipped the first X-ray of Jerome's skull onto the lighted screen. There it was—the bullet. After entering from behind his ear, the bullet had traveled through his sinus and had come to rest in his nasal cavity. It apparently had done very little damage, as his nose wasn't even bleeding.

"Well, I've never seen that before," the doctor stated. With that he asked for a pair of McGill forceps. He inserted the thin forceps into Jerome's left nostril and easily extracted the bullet, which made a clinking sound as it was dropped into an awaiting basin.

If Jerome had had his way, he would have just blown the bullet out of his nose and saved himself several hundreds of dollars' worth of hospital bills.

Communicating with the Spirits

I NEVER BELIEVED IN ghosts—why should I? I was a person firmly planted in reality. The closest I had come to a supernatural event was while I was working a cardiac arrest in the back of the ambulance; the song "Stairway to Heaven" came on the rig radio. It took a heck of a lot for me to become a believer, and there is no one else in the world other than Martin Chwalek who could have taken me on that journey.

It was 1985. After several years of a hiring freeze, a large class of paramedic candidates graduated from the Fire Academy and were dispatched into the field. This led to an excess of fire paramedic/drivers, one of whom was me. I was often extra.

It was decided that extras should ride with their field chief for their twenty-four-hour shift because it would allow the candidates to get some much-needed experience on the ambulance.

Martin Chwalek was my field chief. Martin was weird, really weird. Have you ever been around a person so strange that whenever you are with him, nothing normal happens? With Martin, the simple act of stopping to get a drink at a convenience store would spiral off into some bizarre encounter or event. It was always like that when I was riding with him. I was in familiar surroundings, yet nothing seemed familiar.

As I positioned myself behind the wheel, Martin said, "After rounds, let's head over to 5801 North Pulaski. Did you know it used to be a tuberculosis center?" I opened my mouth to answer what would have been a "no," but I didn't get any further.

"There are underground tunnels that connect the buildings...can't you just picture the TB patients being wheeled through the dark passages, hacking away with bloody phlegm hanging from their chins?" Martin asked with a faraway look in his eye and a sheer excitement that I didn't quite get. My mouth still hung open; I didn't know what to say. Even if I had answered, I don't think Martin would have heard me. He was lost in his tuberculosis reverie.

We headed north on Pulaski, just north of Bryn Mawr toward the entrance to what is now called North Park Village. There was a guard at the gate who paid no attention to us, as we were in a fire department vehicle and seemingly on official business.

North Park Village spans an area from Peterson on the north to Bryn Mawr on the south, and from Pulaski to the west and Central Park to the east. It includes senior citizen housing, a school for the developmentally disabled, a gymnasium and parkland with a nature center encompassing 158 acres. It is the largest city-owned natural area on the North Side of Chicago.

Originally farmland, Chicago grew up around it. In 1911, the city of Chicago bought the land to establish a sanitarium called the Chicago Municipal Tuberculosis Sanitarium, which was one of the largest of its kind in the country. It operated from 1915 through the 1970s. By the 1950s and 1960s, the disease incidence of tuberculosis was drastically reduced through improvements in public hygiene and new medications. The sanitarium became underused by the 1970s and closed in 1974.

Although it was initially slotted for the development of high-rise buildings, the city of Chicago, the Chicago Park District, and various organizations fought over what to do with this huge chunk of land, a third of which had remained in its natural condition. Rich in native grasses, it included an oak savanna, wetland and a pond. Wood ducks, geese, painted turtles, deer and raccoons were frequent inhabitants, as well as foxes, bullfrogs and great blue herons. When Martin and I rolled through the gates, many of the original buildings still stood in a state of suspended animation, their future was still uncertain.

The sanitarium grounds were divided into two sections—the southern part of it had cottages for female patients, and the northern part had a section for the men. East of an administration building were dining halls, one for men, and another for women. There were infirmary buildings with a capacity of three hundred beds. The powerhouse, which provided heat and electricity, lay to the east along with a laundry facility. A church, which still stands today, was centrally located. A morgue, housing for nurses, a garage, a farmhouse and barns were also located on the grounds. The facility had been able to house 650 patients.

I had no idea what Martin thought we could do or find there; the place had long been abandoned. I drove east, passing a small herd of grazing deer. Deer grazing in Chicago, I thought. That's cool. We came upon a large building with a huge smokestack. A car was parked outside.

"Let's go in. Maybe there's someone here who can tell us something about the place." Sure enough, the car belonged to an old-timer who ran the powerhouse, which still provided some heat and electricity to the buildings. He had worked there when the sanitarium was still up and running.

Martin was transfixed by every word the man said and asked question after question. I was only half-listening, wondering when we were going to be on our way.

"Are there really underground tunnels?" he asked.

"Yes, the tunnels connect the main buildings of the sanitarium and were used by the staff to transport laundry and food carts in bad weather."

Martin's eyes lit up. "Can we go into the tunnels?"

"No, the entrances have long been bricked up."

"Are there any buildings we can go into?"

"No, they're in pretty poor condition and are all locked up."

Martin's enthusiasm was not in the least diminished. "Do you mind if we walk around a bit?"

"No, not at all. Ya know, if you want to see one of the original buildings, there is one on your way out. Take the second left and go down a narrow driveway if you want to take a look. It used to be the men's dormitory."

"Thanks!" Martin said.

It was early winter but a warm day for that time of year, so we did a bit of exploring. Walking around the back of the powerhouse, we came upon an old barn, a root cellar and a dilapidated greenhouse. They must have grown and stored their own food, I thought. OK, maybe it was pretty interesting.

Once in our rig, we headed west and took the second left. It was just beginning to get dark as we made our way down a narrow driveway. Massive oak trees loomed over our seemingly tiny vehicle, a few crumbled leaves clung to branches that danced about in a wintery front that had just blown in. Tree limbs lurched back and forth as the driveway disappeared and gave way to a large ancient structure.

It had only two floors, and was much longer than it was tall. I pulled up to the west wing of the building where a door was visible. It was pitch black outside by this time. The sun seemed to have made its escape in record time.

I threw it into "park" and stepped out, my hair flying about in the cold breeze. We walked a short distance to the building and came to a set of glass French doors. Peering into the darkness inside, I couldn't see anything. Martin tried the door. It was locked.

Oh ye of little faith, I thought, apparently you did not have the delinquent upbringing I had. French doors? No problem. As Martin turned and began to walk back toward our vehicle, I grasped each doorknob and pulled them both at the same time with equal force. The doors easily popped open.

Stepping over the threshold into the building, a shroud of darkness engulfed us. I pulled out my penlight. It cast a tiny beam of light that danced about from the floor to the walls to the ceiling. It disappeared down a long hallway directly in front of us that seemed to traverse the entire length of the building. Inching forward, our only guide was my puny beam of light that was cast onto the floor in front of us. After about twenty-five feet we came upon a wooden spiral staircase on our left that led to the second floor. Suddenly, a loud cracking noise echoed throughout the building. We froze in mid-step.

If I were to try to describe the noise, the closest I could come would be the sound a metal baseball bat would make hitting a wooden object. It came from above at the far end of the hallway. It was a deafening sound that marched down the ceiling toward us at regular intervals. It momentarily stopped right at the top of the stairway by where we stood, and then it began to march back down toward the end of the hallway from where it had originated.

I grabbed Martin's arm with both hands and squeezed tight; my heart was pounding in my ears, and I couldn't breathe. I had never been so terrified in all my life. For half a second, I was immobilized, frozen in place.

"Let's get out of here!" I said, still attached to Martin's arm and pulling him as I turned to run out the way we had come in. He was resisting my pull and not cooperating.

"Let's communicate with the spirit," he pleaded.

With all the strength I could muster—which was a lot, as my adrenaline was pumping—I pulled him along out of the building. He hesitantly followed. Once outside, I made for the buggy.

Ripping open the door, I launched myself into the rig, slammed the door and locked it. I felt like my heart was going to explode out of my chest. Martin was out of breath. Maybe he had wanted to communicate with the spirit, but he was also visibly shaken. We sat for a few moments; the only sound was our labored breathing. Martin got out and closed the doors to the building.

Once back in the rig, he said, "Let's get out of here."

We spent the rest of the shift trying to come up with any plausible explanation of what it could have been that we had heard—an explanation for something of this world that is.

"Maybe it was the radiators on the second floor. The old guy said the powerhouse still provided some heat to the building to keep the pipes from freezing. I'm sure they are so old that if they went on they would make a loud noise."

"Yeah, that could explain it," I said. I was desperate to find any explanation for what had happened. A creepy feeling had taken hold of me and would not let go. It was the usual "things are amiss/nothing is normal" feeling I would get when I was with Martin, but it was magnified by about a hundred times. With every explanation we came up with, the funk I was in began to lift.

"Maybe there's a homeless guy living up there who was trying to scare us," I said.

"Yes, that is definitely a possibility."

We both knew without a doubt that we had to return to find the answer. On our next work day, Martin made sure I was extra and riding with him. We decided to go back at the exact same time of day to try to recreate the scenario. This time I was determined to find an answer as to what had caused that noise.

After pulling open the French doors, with my penlight in hand, we began to explore the building a little further. Directly to our left was what appeared to be a sitting room. We took a detour from the hallway and walked around the room. Shining the light here and there, we commented on the fireplace and lovely woodwork.

There's nothing here to fear, I thought. The more we wandered about, the more confident and lighthearted I became. Heading back to the hallway, we made our way just as we had during our previous shift. The spiral staircase was directly on our left when it happened. Down came the noise from the end of the hallway ceiling.

"Crack, crack, crack!" The noise stopped directly overhead at the top of the stairs. I had a death grip on Martin's arm. This time he began to pull away and run for the door. Fighting every instinct to flee with him, I took a firmer grip on his arm and pulled him up the stairway toward the noise. Our chests heaving, we stopped at the top of the stairs with our backs glued to the wall.

I was expecting something, although I had no idea what that might have been. What we saw was absolutely nothing. After several minutes of immobilization, we caught our breath. Hesitantly, on guard for anything that could have caused that terrifying noise, we began to search the second floor.

The radiators were cold. There was no sign of human or animal life. Even if someone had been trying to hide and scare us, it would have been impossible not to be heard throughout the building when walking about. The floor was littered with small pieces of plaster that had fallen from the ceiling and they made a crunching sound with every step we took. The sound we had heard had definitely not been a crunching sound from someone walking on the plaster. After making our way back to the rig, we sat in silence. We were out of ideas.

I took the next few days to reflect on our experience. I was rattled. I had always believed that what you see is what you get and that things are exactly as they appear to be—that everything has an explanation. As hard as we wanted to find one, there was no explanation for what had happened. A shift in my thinking was taking place. The only conclusion I could come to was that there are some things in this world that we can never understand. I found this to be quite unsettling, but I eventually accepted it wholeheartedly.

Clint Dawson, another field chief, was the only guy on the job I felt I could tell this story to—the only one who would not think I was nuts. A week later he told me he had gone to the building, stepped inside, and set out on the exact same walk down the hallway that Martin and I had taken. Nothing had happened.

Given the same set of circumstances, I am certain my close encounter would never have occurred without Martin. Shortly after our adventure, out of the blue, Martin up and quit the job. This really didn't surprise anyone, as he had always walked to the beat of a different drummer. I will never know the impact that experience had on him, if it had any at all. I was sent back to my assignment and I never saw Martin again. For me, it ended up having a much deeper meaning—it was more than just a strange encounter.

My eyes were opened to a pattern of events in my life that anyone else might have looked upon as random; but for me, when seen as a whole, with my new insight, they could not possibly have been.

Many people cannot see the path that is set out before them. I was more open to the "seeing" part of my life that I had not taken into account before my ghost encounter. It is trusting in the fact that there are things I don't understand, but if I paid attention, my path in life would eventually reveal itself. As for Martin: He left Chicago for some land he owned in Mississippi. Last I heard, he had become a minister.

The Wrench

"AMBULANCE 15, TAKE the injured victim at the construction site at 5962 West Chicago Avenue." Mike and I pulled up to a four-story building that was just a skeleton of metal beams. Several construction workers were waving us over. They stood in a semicircle some distance away from an injured coworker who was lying on his back on the ground. As we approached, they silently pointed in unison at our patient.

I kneeled down next to him and asked, "What happened to ya?"

"I really don't know. I think something hit me on the head."

"Did you have a hard hat on?"

"No."

"Psst, psst." One of his coworkers was discreetly trying to get my attention. As I spoke with him, my partner, Mike, checked our patient's vital signs. In a hushed voice, so his injured friend would not hear, he explained to me what had happened.

"I was about three stories up when that lug wrench," he paused and pointed to a large wrench lying on the ground a few feet away from the patient— "fell out of my back pocket. It went in."

"What do you mean 'went in'?"

"The handle of the wrench went straight into the top of his head."

"How far in did it go?"

"It looked like about four inches, then he fell over and the wrench came out."

I immediately went to the patient's side and parted the hair on the top of his head. Sure enough, there it was—a large laceration that had not been visible because there was no bleeding. I took my partner aside and explained the situation.

Our ward was alert and had a grayish pallor to his skin. I had no idea if he knew what had happened, and he didn't ask. I could't see the point in telling him, as it would have been counterproductive to upset him and possibly cause his blood pressure to skyrocket.

"Just stay there and don't move. We'll be right back," I told our patient. We shifted into high gear.

After grabbing the stretcher, cervical collar and backboard, we loaded him into the rig. I started an IV and applied the heart monitor as my partner gave him some oxygen.

"What's your name? What's your address? Do you have any medical problems?" At first, our patient, John, answered all of my questions in an appropriate manner.

"Do you have pain anywhere?"

"Well, my head sandwich dog leash." As he spoke these words, he looked stunned. I could tell by the confused look on his face that he could hear what he was saying and knew it made no sense.

Aphasia is the loss of the ability to understand or express speech. It is caused by brain damage. John had sustained damage to the part of his brain that is responsible for speech. He could, however, understand everything I said, but he could not express himself verbally.

I have had many patients with brain damage caused by gunshot wounds, a blow to the head, or a stroke. In every instance, the patient had been either unconscious or confused to the point that he didn't know what was going on. Our patient, on the other hand, knew what was going on. He could hear himself speaking but had no control over the words that came out of his mouth. How frightening that must have been for him.

I chose not to ask John any more questions and instead reassured him that we would be at the hospital soon. A silent pact had been made between us, as I knew by the look in his eyes that he was terrified to utter another word.

We were en route to Loyola Medical Center, a Level 1 Trauma Center. I delivered a report to the hospital on the way. Once in the ED, we slid John onto the hospital gurney. The trauma team descended upon him and immediately whisked him off to surgery.

I have been on thousands of runs, most of which I have forgotten. However, occasionally a run will stick with me, and this one did. I often thought about John, recalling the look of terror in his eyes. I wondered if the damage to his brain would be permanent.

A few weeks later, my field chief delivered a letter from John's parents to my partner and I. They thanked us for taking care of their son and for transporting him to a trauma center where he was able to receive the best treatment for his serious injury. He was still in the intensive care unit but was expected to enter rehab in the near future.

Don's Story

"**D**O YOU HAVE a cigarette?"

For the record, the last cigarette I smoked was outside of Resurrection Hospital Emergency Department after Don Burke dropped dead.

In 1992, I put in for a transfer to Ambulance 20, which is also the home of Engine 86 and Truck 57. The firehouse is located in the Belmont Heights neighborhood, which is known as the "HIP" for the shopping district on the corner of Harlem and Irving Park Avenues called the Harlem Irving Plaza.

Walking into a new assignment for the first time is always an adventure. The fire department is like a big family—everyone talks. There is a saying in the department: "Telephone, telegraph, tell a fireman." I have worked some thirty years in an atmosphere of ninety-nine percent men. Ladies, there are some things I could tell you about men that you would never want to know, but that is for another time. What I will divulge is that men gossip.

When a spot at a firehouse becomes vacant, there is nonstop speculation as to who will put in for it. This can go on for months without anyone ever asking the prospective candidates if they are actually putting in for a transfer to the assignment.

The reason for the ongoing gossip is a vicious cycle of non-communication. No one will ask anyone if they put in because that would be communicating, which is an unmanly act, reminiscent of high treason. In effect, this causes the gossip to continue until a transfer order comes out.

I was once privy to a conversation between several firefighters speculating on whether a particular officer had put in for a vacant position at the firehouse.

"Why don't you just ask him if he put in?" I suggested. All heads turned in my direction, mouths agape, as if I were speaking a strange and foreign language. A long silence followed, and they quickly changed the subject as if they had not heard the words I had uttered.

Walking into my new assignment for the first time was going to be quite a treat. I knew exactly what had been going on for the last several months. Word gets around of the possible candidates likely to bid on the vacant assignment. Gossip of every type is brought into the mix. Anything anyone had ever heard, speculated about, or just made up about a person is brought to the table. Then the day comes when you walk through the kitchen door, the heart of the firehouse.

The screen door creaked as I wrenched it open and it slammed shut behind me. I grabbed my plate and found my way into line to get some lunch. In front of me were two firefighters, Don and Jack. They were in their late fifties and riding out the end of their careers on Engine 86. The engine was slow, only in need of a light dusting and an occasional changing of its square tires. It was the perfect spot to spend the twilight years of a firefighter's career.

Don and Jack resembled Tweedle Dee and Tweedle Dum. They were about the same height and girth, their belts slug low, disappearing under identical keg-shaped bellies. When they turned around and introduced themselves, Don added, "We have dicky do."

"What's dicky do?" I asked.

"Our stomachs stick out more than our dickies do."

I had to laugh and knew that this was the place for me.

Don and I immediately hit it off. He frequented a pub on Belmont Avenue and asked me to join him for a few pints of black and tan on an off day; now that was right up my alley. Don's daughter Patti and his wife, Rosemary, were at the firehouse often. Patti had kids a bit older than mine and would give me much-appreciated hand-me-downs.

Don had some, let's say, unhealthy habits. He smoked about four packs of unfiltered cigarettes a day. Eating was high adventure, delving into grease and fat; on his plate, the vegetable and fruit were uninvited guests.

We all slept in the same bunkroom. The only privacy I had was a small wall built around my bed. Don's snoring sounded like a flock of geese on a cross continental migration. I had, however, worked out a technique for getting some rest. I would insert earplugs and get into bed well before he came up to the bunkroom. If I was in a deep sleep by the time he began his nighttime follies, it was all good.

More often than not, we would get a few runs in the middle of the night. Upon my return to the bunkroom, I would listen to Don's distinctive snore, letting my mind wander as I wished for a few minutes of uninterrupted sleep. I sometimes drifted off and had a reoccurring dream about Don.

In my dream, it was the morning and the guys were shaking me to consciousness because Don had died in his sleep. I ran to his bunk and found that it was too late—he had been dead too long. I had this dream quite often. I tried to stop it, as it was really gruesome to think of someone I knew dying. I had never had to work on anyone I knew and did not want to find out what that would involve, but he was such a terrible physical specimen. What if the worst should happen?

At two in the morning, we were returning from a call. After cruising up onto the firehouse apron, I stopped the rig and let my partner, Jimmy, out. He entered the firehouse to open the overhead door. I swung out onto Harlem Avenue preparing to back the rig in. As I glanced in the sideview mirror, I noticed the engine and truck were out. That was highly unusual. I was putting it in reverse when dispatch beckoned.

"Ambulance 20, take the firefighter down at 7654 West Forest Preserve Drive." Dispatch was famous for giving us as little information as humanly possible. For instance, they would give us a call for a bleeding victim. The victim could be bleeding from a paper cut or from a butcher knife to the chest. Every run was like the surprise party I never wanted. Over the years, I learned it was better not to ask; just go and deal with whatever it was when we got there.

As we approached the scene, it was clear the guys had been fighting a fire.

"Don's down, Don's down!" Mike yelled as we pulled up. It was very dark and there was a lot of mud caused by runoff from water that had been thrown on the fire.

It was difficult to even see him at first. Don was laying on his back in the muck, a firefighter was doing CPR.

"What happened?"

"He put on his SCBA, (self-contained breathing apparatus), fell over backwards and arrested." CPR had been started immediately.

"Let's move him to the rig," Jimmy said. Our only course of action for the moment was to continue CPR and to ventilate via bag-valve mask, as we couldn't see a thing.

Once in the ambulance, I hooked Don up to the heart monitor. It wasn't good. He was in V-fib. Ventricular fibrillation is the heart improvising, ad-libbing a jig instead of doing the fox trot. It means that very little blood is being circulated to the body, and most importantly, to the brain. We juiced up the defibrillator and zapped Don several times, incrementally increasing the amount of joules delivered. His heart would just not convert to a normal rhythm. Jimmy immediately intubated, inserting a breathing tube into his trachea as I slipped an IV into his vein. We continued CPR as we gave him medications to make his heart more likely to convert to a normal rhythm. We defibrillated several more times with no luck.

I could hear my heart pounding in my ears; my worst nightmare had come to light. I got behind the wheel, flipped on the emergency lights and siren and headed for Resurrection Hospital.

Jimmy informed Resurrection we were on the way and relayed his report of our treatment thus far. He continued working en route and commanded a firefighter for assistance. We delivered Don to the emergency department; we were still unable to restore a normal heart rhythm. As we slid him onto a hospital gurney, a mass of doctors and nurses converged upon him.

Not knowing what to do with myself, I crept into the stockroom to replace all the equipment we had used. It was better to keep busy than to mull over what had just occurred. I had never heard of anyone coming back after such an extended period of time without a viable heart rhythm. If they did somehow restore a heartbeat, Don would most likely have brain damage.

I felt we did everything we could have done for him. At the hospital they continued to work. I stayed out of sight as battalion chiefs, deputy commissioners and the fire department priest, Father Mulcrone, arrived. I couldn't face his family, who I'm sure had been alerted of the situation by that time.

Outside the emergency department, in the ambulance bay, I smoked a cigarette I had bummed off of another paramedic. "This cigarette tastes like crap," I thought and tossed it. I stepped back into the emergency department.

I expected to hear the sad news that Don had been pronounced dead; however, that was not to be. I could hear Patti speaking to her father in a hushed and desperate voice, "Come on Dad! Come on Dad!" I peeked behind the curtain and saw a huge ball of EKG paper gathered on the floor and Don's daughter at his side.

"What's happening?" I whispered to one of the nurses.

"We keep getting him back and then losing him."

Jimmy and I slunk out to the ambulance and returned to quarters. We were not in the least convinced that the outcome would be anything but grim. It had just been too long. Back at quarters, the whole house was put out of service. We all sat at the kitchen table in silence staring at the walls as the sun rose. Now and then a chief would come with news.

"They got him back and he is stable for now."

"He is being transferred to the ICU."

"He's going for bypass surgery because every artery in his heart is completely blocked."

Bypass surgery? Don could not possibly survive surgery after everything he had been through, I thought. My seven A.M. relief arrived, and I went home.

Later that day, I called Resurrection Hospital and inquired as to Don's condition. He had made it through surgery and was in the surgical intensive care unit. I immediately headed over to the hospital. Don's family was gathered in the waiting area. His daughter Patti shared the story of what had occurred the morning Don had left for his shift.

She had asked her dad if he could give her money for gas. He gruffly replied that he had no money. When she arrived at the hospital, they gave her Don's wallet. In it, she was surprised to find two hundred dollars. As Don drifted between life and death, she had whispered in his ear... "Dad—I have your wallet."

It was time to go see the patient. I entered Don's room and saw that he was tied to his bed, pulling with all his strength at the restraints. For a few seconds, recognition seemed to come to his unseeing eyes, even though he had not yet regained consciousness. He smiled a crooked smile, which was all he could muster with a breathing tube in place, and then continued to fight some unseen foe.

"Is he sedated?" I asked the nurse.

"Yes. It isn't working."

The next day, Don recognized his wife, Rosemary. From then on, he continued to improve, eventually making a full recovery. He remembered everything up until they got the call for the fire.

Don Burke lived many more years in retirement—long enough to see four grandchildren born. He often came to the firehouse to visit. I will never know how Don made it through that ordeal without any brain damage. Strong and timely CPR must have been the key. But CPR cannot circulate nearly as much oxygenated blood to the body as a properly beating heart can. In the short term it is effective if the heart can be restored to a normal rhythm within a timely manner. Don's ordeal had lasted more than forty-five minutes.

My husband's take on the whole situation was simple. He said that Don's brain probably thought he was taking a long drag on a cigarette.

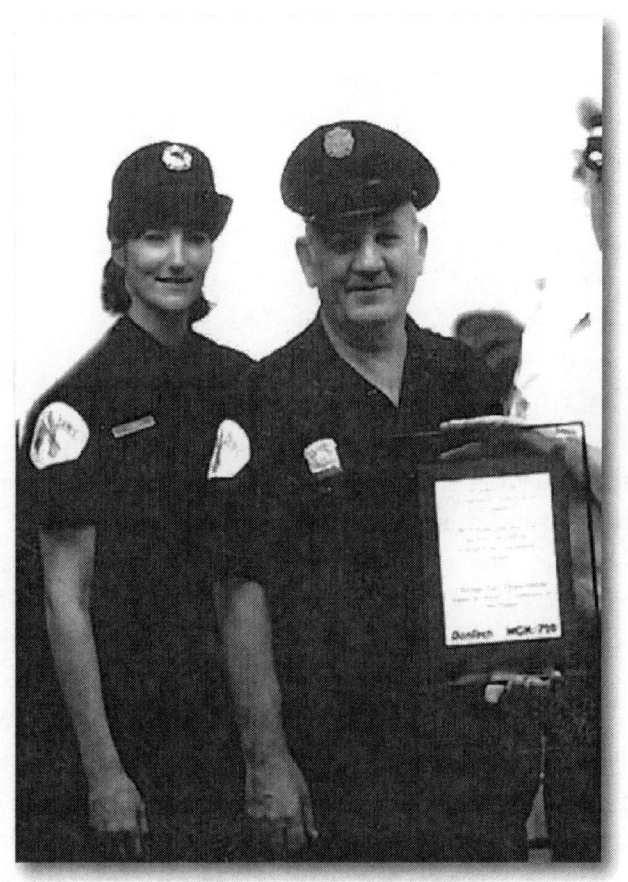

Don after his recovery in 1992

Badge of Honor

IN THE EARLY 1980s, the Chicago Fire Department Emergency Medical Service, or EMS, was a small operation. There had been a hiring freeze in effect for several years. Without an influx of new candidates, everybody knew everybody. This was a time before the ambulance assist program, which was implemented in the 1990s. Today, an assist fire company is dispatched with an ambulance on almost every run for the purposes of manpower.

"Manpower" could include anything from carrying equipment and assisting with patient conveyance, to helping out with patient care like CPR. But in the '80s, we were on our own. Loaded down with equipment on our backs like pack mules, we would often have to carry a patient down several flights of stairs. When we worked a cardiac arrest, during which many hands were needed, we called for a second ambulance instead of a fire company as we do today. The fire companies were not in the mix of ambulance runs unless we had an extremely large patient, which was rare back in the day.

Paramedics looked out for each other and tried not to let another ambulance take any of their runs. That was sometimes impossible, as several calls could come in at the same time into one area. But we did our best to monitor the radio and step it up at the hospital when it became busy.

Taking care of ones district was our unwritten code—our badge of honor. After so many years and so many new people, our badge of honor seemed to go by the wayside. One paramedic in particular chose to completely disregard this code of conduct.

IT'S NOT THE TRAUMA, IT'S THE DRAMA

In 2003, I was a paramedic in charge assigned to Ambulance 7, which is located in the Belmont Gardens neighborhood. We were getting hammered with run after run, as was everyone else that day. It was about eight in the evening, dinner at the firehouse had since gone cold and shriveled and was sitting in a foil-covered plate in the kitchen awaiting our untimely return.

We pulled into West Suburban Hospital and backed in next to Ambulance 23, a West Side rig located at Engine 113's quarters. We delivered our patient to the emergency department, and then chit-chatted with the guys on Ambulance 23 as I finished my report. Greg, the paramedic in charge on Ambulance 23, was a large chap who wore a raccoon hat in summer and winter. His hat was not regulation.

Both ambulances rolled out of the hospital bay at the same time. We turned north on Austin Boulevard. Ambulance 23, along with Greg and his raccoon hat, turned south as we headed back to our respective quarters, each informing dispatch we were on the return.

A few minutes later, dispatch called. "Ambulance 23." No answer.

"Ambulance 23, Ambulance 23." Still no answer.

"Ambulance 7."

"7 go," I replied.

"Take the sick person at 5324 West Harrison."

"Wow, that's like a block away from Ambulance 23's quarters," mentioned Jason, my candidate partner for the day.

"Yes it is, yes it is."

I gave it a few seconds, trying to give Greg the benefit of the doubt, hoping he would answer dispatch and take his run. I sent a message via computer in an effort to spur him into action.

"Where are you?" My message kindly inquired.

"Austin and Jackson," he answered. He was already back in his area. My head felt like it was going to explode. What was he doing? Did I actually have to do this? Had he left his badge of honor at home?

"Dispatch is calling you for a run by your firehouse," I typed. No answer.

We took the patient to Loretto Hospital, which was just down the street from Ambulance 23's quarters. I was calm, I was quiet. I was on a mission. I was not sure what that mission was, but it was going to be something.

"Hey Jason, swing by Ambulance 23's quarters."

The firehouse is a small old single-engine house; the ambulance must have been an afterthought. It is absurdly smashed into the tiny quarters next to the engine. For that reason, paramedics sometimes left the ambulance parked outside the firehouse. And yes, Ambulance 23 was parked outside.

I approached the rig and tried the driver's side door. Amazingly, it was open, and the rig was running. Ambulances were stolen more often than you would imagine. The ensuing charges, suspension and paperwork were usually enough of a deterrent to keep the rig locked up.

I eased the rig into gear and cruised a half-block east and parked it in front of a large Dumpster. The ambulance was not visible from the vantage point of the firehouse.

After slamming it into "park", I was about to exit—but wait, what luck—the hat! Greg's raccoon hat was perched on the dash. I slapped it on my head, locked the ambulance doors and made for my rig at a fast clip. I vaulted into the passenger seat, out of breath with excitement at my stroke of luck.

"Back to quarters, Jeeves," I said in my best British accent.

"You can't do that!"

"Oh yes I can." Jason did not look well. In fact, he looked terrified probably because it was his second day on the job. Well, he was learning a very valuable lesson.

As we made our way back to quarters, I asked Jason if he had a cell phone.

"Yeah," he said.

"Can I borrow it?"

"Sure."

I checked the computer every few seconds to see when Ambulance 23 got their next run. I knew I wouldn't have to wait long, as they were a busy rig. Their next call appeared on our screen. I dialed their quarters.

"Engine 113's quarters."

"Oh, hi. If the guys on the ambulance come back in because they can't find their rig, tell them it's parked in front of the Dumpster." And then I hung up.

Ah, how sweet it would have been to see the look on their faces when they stepped outside and discovered nothing but a lot of air where their rig had been. I can only imagine...

We soon received a barrage of messages on our computer from Ambulance 23. They were all quite long, the tone was unfriendly. I didn't read any of them, delete-delete-delete. I was in a fantastic mood and did not want to have it ruined by ill will. I wore the raccoon hat for the remainder of the shift, proudly flaunting my spoils. We didn't run into them for the rest of the night.

The next workday, I felt I should return Greg's hat. I strolled into his quarters, wearing the hat, of course. He was sitting in the kitchen. I removed the hat from my head and gently placed it on the table in front of him.

"Sorry, but we were really hungry and hadn't had dinner," he said.

Oh, Lord. I hope the gods of the unwritten code hadn't heard that. He deserved his badge of honor ripped from his chest.

"Oh, I know, everyone was really busy. Sorry I took your hat." (Translation—you can't be serious? And we weren't hungry too?)

Greg never brought the event up again, but I will tell you this—on every run after his ambulance had mysteriously disappeared, that guy hauled ass.

La Tortuga

It was my first day as the ambulance commander on Ambulance 34. There had not been a commander there for over five years because no one was insane enough to put in for the spot. The ambulance was crazy busy, the firehouse a structure of ancient origins; it had not aged gracefully. I had been mandatorily assigned there for "the good of the department" and had to stay for a minimum of one year.

"Telephone, telegraph, tell a firemen" was in full swing. One by one, they sidled up to me, speaking in low voices with a look of concern on their faces.

"You have to do something about him."

"He needs training."

I had never heard firefighters so concerned about a paramedic.

I knew nothing about my partner other than his name and what the firefighters had discreetly relayed to me. It would be a long twenty-four-hour shift if we didn't hit off —or worse, if we didn't get along at all. Working together at all hours of the day and night, we are thrown into all sorts of bizarre and sometimes dangerous situations. Working with someone you understand and you know understands you is like a gift. It can turn an exhausting, mostly thankless job into a fun and stress-free shift.

After my first glance at my new partner, Eduardo, for no reason other than a gut feeling, I knew that it would be OK.

Eddie was tall and thin, with thick glasses and dark shaggy hair. He was about ten years younger than I was and had about fifteen years less seniority. He was a new guy, with only a couple of years on the job. Colombian in origin, he spoke Spanish, which would come in handy in the heavily Mexican neighborhood of Little Village. Everything about Eduardo was slow. He walked, talked and in general functioned at the pace of a turtle, hence his nickname, *La Tortuga*.

    A snail plods along. Like anything else, a snail can be in a hurry and exert itself, but could you tell? I don't think so. Eddie, on the other hand, could give the illusion of exerting himself, even when he wasn't moving any faster than usual, like a turtle whose legs were pumping away, yet not really getting anywhere. It took some time to figure out how he accomplished this feat. Upon close observation, he would make some sudden grandiose move, as if he had just done something extremely strenuous, adding a huge sigh or grunt. But in fact he really hadn't done anything at all, or had not done anything more than I had done. For example, while conveying someone down the stairs on a stair chair (a little chair on wheels), he would complain under his breath about the extreme weight of the patient and commence to grunt and groan. I believe he could even make himself perspire. I would be at the top of the chair, and Eddie would be at the bottom.

    "Ed, she only weighs ninety pounds."

    Eduardo had a relaxed demeanor and was a man of few words. In fact, he said so few words that I sometimes felt the urge to poke him with a stick to make sure he was awake. It was this manner of appearing to be in a stupor that had caused the firefighters to be so concerned.

    Day or night, as soon as we got back to the firehouse, he would doze off in a chair. When the firefighters did their chores, they sometimes had to sweep around him. Now this is OK on one level, as the ambulance was much busier than the engine or truck. The paramedics didn't have any assigned housework because we were out for almost the entire shift. On the other hand, if one were to jump in and do the simplest thing, like wipe off the dinner table or help scrub out the apparatus floor, it would be a show of camaraderie. The guys would tell him to stop, yet he should continue. Chances are that before he could do much more than pick up a squeegee, we would get a run anyway. Eddie apparently had never picked up on these rules of firehouse conduct. So, I had to ask.

"Ed, do you ever try to help out with housework?"

"No."

"Just try to help out. We will probably get a run before you can actually do much anyway."

"OK."

Eddie was all over it.

As I crawled into bed at four A.M., I begged the ambulance gods to grant me five minutes of rest. I cranked my electric blanket to broil. The drafty bunkroom was freezing, just the way the guys liked it. The window at the far end of the room was wide open, snow drifted in as a fan blew the flakes about. The firefighters all slept soundly, in boxers with only a sheet covering them.

An electric blanket is a must in winter and summer—summer is almost worse as the air conditioner is cranked to the meat locker setting. Whenever a fuse was blown in that decrepit building, they would blame me and my electric blanket.

"Ambulance 34, take the overdose"... so much for my five minutes. The ambulance gods were frowning upon me. I dragged myself out of my warm nest and gingerly made my way down the iron spiral staircase, which was more of a death trap than a means of conveyance.

Any normal partner would have met me in the ambulance; however, I did not have a normal partner. I made for the TV room on the first floor. The door creaked open. It was pitch black in there. Outlines of forms were visible on the couches. I knew which one was Eduardo's and shook him until he awoke.

"Come on, we have a run."

"What? What?"

"We have a run. Let's go."

After a few workdays of having to wake Eddie up for every run after midnight,

I had to ask.

"So why don't you wake up at night? Do you not hear the bells, or do you hear them and think it's a dream or what?"

"I'm not sure."

"Well, don't worry about it, just as long as I know where you are, that's fine. I'll come and get you." After that, I never had to wake up Eddie again. On every call after midnight, I would find him already waiting in the ambulance; it was fascinating.

On runs, Eduardo had some interesting habits. One was that he would not unfold the stair chair spontaneously for any reason. I had to ask him to open it every time. The patient could be unconscious and lying in a pool of blood on the floor and he would stand there with folded chair in hand. So, I had to ask.

"Why don't you ever open the chair?"

"Maybe there is a chance we won't need it."

"How about you just open it when we need it."

"OK."

That was that. It never happened again. Eddie also had the habit of moving at "La Tortuga" pace after we pulled up to the scene of a run.

"*Mum, why do they call it a run? No one is running,*" asked my daughter once while visiting the firehouse. I like to make it from the ambulance to the patient's door in a timely manner, but she is right, there is no running going on here. If you ever see paramedics running, you best run too as something is dangerously amiss.

Because I was in the passenger seat, I had a shorter distance to the side door compartments that contained the two essential pieces of equipment that we brought in on every call—the jump bag, or QRB (quick response bag) and the stair chair. I would grab the bag, Ed would grab the chair. After several workdays of finding myself alone at the patient's door while Eduardo was still grappling with the stair chair completely out of sight on the far side of the ambulance. I had to ask.

"Eddie, I could have been killed in ten different ways by the time you got to the door. Can we go together?"

"OK."

From then on, Eddie was always at my side.

On calls, when we had a sick person to tend to, Eduardo was quite competent in his skills, but even when he was cranked into high gear, he operated at a frustratingly sluggish pace. I had to do something to get him moving when I needed some action. I did find a way to get him into gear, but it would be used sparingly, as it involved him transforming into a superhero. You wouldn't summon Superman if you needed a jar opened. He would be called upon only in a dire emergency. That's the way it went with Eddie.

When we were returning from a call at three in the morning, I asked: "Hey Ed, what's your middle name?"

"I will never tell you."

"Just give me a hint."

"It begins with an A."

"Arthur," "No." "Andy," "No." "Antonio," "No." "Aaron," "No." "Alexander," "No."

One week later, four A.M., "Amos," "No." "Adam," "No." "Angus," "No."

Next workday, while restraining a berserk patient: "Arturo, Anthony."

"No and no!"

We had a call for a fifty-year-old male, a psych patient, at five-thirty in the morning. We had been going all day and night on run after run. I was fully functional, but my brain had entered another dimension that defied time and space.

Exiting the ambulance, we found our patient at the curb. He was an unkempt, somewhat odorous male who smelled strongly of alcohol. I opened the side door and he stepped up and took a seat on the bench. He told me he had been drinking for many days and had been seeing things and hearing voices.

Eddie was outside by the curb, softly conversing in Spanish with the patient's daughter. "She said that her father has been drinking for three days and is now hallucinating."

"Yes, I know. He told me."

Eddie stared at me, slightly baffled. "He only speaks Spanish."

I speak rudimentary Spanish at best and understand even less, yet I understood everything the patient had told me. I had entered some kind of altered state.

Eduardo hopped up to check our patient's vital signs. He sat next to him and pumped up the blood pressure cuff.

"Armando."

The pumping momentarily stopped. I got it.

I don't really recall how it came to be, but when I would say "Armando," Ed would transform—tights, cape, giant A on his chest. He was able to perform feats of amazing strength and speed. It was like having control of a genie in a bottle.

We had a large lady in the stair chair. She had twisted her ankle in the park and was unable to walk. Unfortunately, we had to wheel her across a football field of grass and dirt to get back to the ambulance. The chair was not rolling well. It constantly needed to be lifted up, tugged and pulled from the bottom as the wheels kept getting stuck in the soft grass and dirt. Our only other option was for us both to carry the stair chair, which would have been exhausting. After a few minutes of tugging and lifting, I had had enough.

"Armando!"

Tights and cape appeared, muscles bulged, super hero music began to play. Armando spun the chair around so it was facing backwards. Facing forwards, he began pulling the chair instead of both of us pushing it. Off he sprinted at a super human-speed with the chair in tow, leaving me in the dust and the patient's hair flying in the breeze.

"I'm dying for a tamale. Let's stop at La Familia." I suggested. It was my favorite Mexican restaurant. The tamal de pollo was fabulous. I could just picture the little Mexican grandma in the back rolling them. The only problem was that they often ran out of them.

The paramedic in charge (PIC) of Ambulance 19, had also discovered the La Familia's chicken tamales. We pulled up outside the restaurant; Ambulance 19 was already parked out front. Damn!

I got in line behind the PIC of 19. "Hey, how's it going?" I asked her.

"Great, how's your day?"

"Pretty decent so far." I said.

"What are you getting?" I inquired.

"Chicken tamales."

Damn!

"I'll have six chicken tamales," the PIC of Ambulance 19 said.

"We only have three left."

"I'll take them." She glanced back at me before making her escape. "Sorry!"

I was devastated. Eddie suggested that I just get something else. He felt so bad for me that he even insisted on buying. Reluctantly, I took his suggestion, but it just wasn't the same.

At three in the morning, I found out just how much it wasn't the same. I came down with a case of food poisoning. Nausea and stomach cramps do not go well with being up all night hauling people around. In fact, I was sicker than most of our patients. By four A.M., I was in agony. I either needed to lay-up and go home or somehow make it until my seven A.M. relief would come in. It was absurd to lay-up at that hour.

Laying up involved signing into an emergency department, being examined and getting a doctor's note that stated I couldn't work. I would then have to go back to the firehouse, drive home and call the medical division in the morning. After stuffing myself into my itchy dress uniform, with my doctor's note in tow, I would have to drive downtown to our medical division at the crack of dawn so as not to get stuck in traffic, and then sit in a hot room for several hours before seeing a doctor who may or may not release me for duty. No, I had to make it for just a few more hours. That is how Code Cansado was born. "Cansado" means very tired, and "code" for, well, just because it sounded good. I had the idea of how I could get some rest; Eddie came up with the name. It was a joint effort.

While working on the South Side, I was horrified to learn of a method used to gain some undeserved downtime: letting the ambulances around you pick up the slack. The "to hospital" button on the computer in the ambulance was not pushed until one had been at the hospital for about half an hour, and then the "at hospital" button would be pushed. The perpetrator would get an easy hour or more at the hospital, and dispatch probably wouldn't catch on to what they had done. I decided that that was what we had to do. I told Eduardo that Code Cansado must be used sparingly—only if we were in the direst of straits—and that he must never tell anyone about it. By sleeping on and off in the back of the rig, I made it through the rest of the shift and thanked Eddie for poisoning me.

Our next work day, Eddie was asked to be an acting paramedic in charge. Occasionally there was a shortage of PIC's. Instead of rehiring a paramedic in charge on overtime, they would ask an FPM, (a fire paramedic/driver, which was Eduardo's rank) to act as a PIC. Eddie was to work on Ambulance 19, one of our sister ambulances.

The crews on the ambulances around you can make or break your shift. One guy in your area who's a "dog" can throw a monkey wrench into the works. Luckily, we had a tight-knit group and we all did our best to take our runs. Ambulance 19 was to our south, and to our west was Ambulance 10.

Ambulance 10 was the cool ambulance to our geek ambulance. They always had some awesome run. I recall wheeling an elderly lady into Mount Sinai Hospital; her complaint was constipation for three days.

As we made our way from the ambulance toward the ED entrance, the guys on Ambulance 10 blew past us, stretcher in tow, with a guy who had a ten-inch butcher knife sticking out of his back. The knife was bandaged in place just like the picture in the paramedic book whose caption read, "never remove an impaled object. It can cause severe hemorrhage; bandage it in place."

The next workday, Ed was the acting PIC on Ambulance 19. I knew I didn't have to worry as I had taught him well. If everyone holds up his or her end, you can generally get a couple of hours of sleep at night, as the volume of calls somewhat decreases. You can still get hammered, but knowing they're your own runs makes it a bit more tolerable.

Sometime after midnight, I noticed the green message light on our computer screen was lit up. I hit the button. The message was from Ambulance 19.

"Code Cansado is in effect."

The return message: "I will kill you."

In the evening, when I was finishing up the paperwork at the hospital, Ed would go out to the ambulance. Reclining in the driver's seat, he would take a nap.

As I stepping out of Saint Anthony Hospital, I was met by the cool evening air. The moon was glowing over Douglas Park. During the day, it was such a bustling and noisy place, but at night it was unnaturally peaceful and quiet. There wasn't a sound to be heard—it was a stillness that rarely comes to the city. I made my way the short distance to the ambulance, which was parked in the bay. I grasped the passenger side door handle. It grumbled a soft metallic creak as it swung open. Apparently Eddie had a problem with his head bobbing as he fell asleep, so he had made a most practical decision. There was La Tortuga, sitting in the driver's seat, sleeping with a cervical collar on. That is how I will always remember my partner.

A little side note on Eddie: While working at his current assignment, he rescued three victims who were trapped against a break wall in Lake Michigan's chop. He swam out several times to rescue each person with total disregard for his own safety. This superhero-like feat earned him the Chicago Fire Department's highest award given to paramedics for bravery and valor in the course of their duty. Way to go, Ed. Armando is alive and well.

The Old Quarters of Ambulance 34

I LOVE A RICKETY old firehouse; it is a silent observer of firehouse life. Working in a building for twenty-four hours, you come to know it more intimately than your own home. Within its walls, members and crews have come and gone, firefighters and paramedics have moved on, and in some cases, passed on.

I first worked Ambulance 34 in 1983 as a candidate paramedic, the bottom of the food chain in our chain of command. In 2005, I returned as the ambulance commander, the highest rank of a paramedic working on an ambulance. After all those years, so many things had changed, yet the firehouse remained exactly as I had left it. With its ancient fixtures and eccentricities, it was like a crusty old friend welcoming me back. I felt a sense of comfort, as I knew this place so well. It has left me with fond memories of its shortcomings, and feelings of nostalgia that a new firehouse cannot muster.

There is a brand new firehouse now, equipped with all the modern conveniences. It's located at 2343 South Kedzie, but in the day, when I first worked on Ambulance 34 in the early 1980s, the old house had character to spare.

Set on a corner in a residential area in the bustling Mexican neighborhood known as Little Village, where three-story brownstones stand shoulder to shoulder, sat the old quarters of Engine 109, Truck 32 and Ambulance 34, located at 2358 South Whipple Street. Firefighters and paramedics were not its only residents. Fleas, mice and rats graced this lovely ancient structure. There were also two sets of gleaming brass fire poles.

Fire poles are no longer used in the modern firehouses for several reasons; the main reason is that the door covering the hole in the second floor to accommodate the pole can be a hazard if left open. It's a two-hinged wooden structure built into the floor that closed around the hole so an innocent person on the second floor in a dark bunkroom taking a walk to the bathroom would not unexpectedly end up on the cement apparatus floor below with several fractured limbs. Occasionally the trapdoor was left open, and the express route to the first floor was taken one too many times.

As we all know, guys will be guys. All sorts of fun can be had with fire poles—sliding down headfirst, no arms, or one leg slides. Severe injuries occurred; such as cracking open of heads and splintering of bones.

Imagine a fire in the middle of the night: Firefighters are snoring away in the bunkroom in a state of unconscious bliss when the bell sounds. Snapped from slumber and jolted awake, they open the trapdoor and quickly slide down the pole to reach their assigned apparatus to save lives, but, just as importantly, to beat the next closest engine or truck company to the fire. Testosterone is pumping; your reputation is on the line. If you don't get there first and the second company beats you into your fire, all will be lost.

Down the pole the men slide. Do you imagine that the guy at the top waits for the guy at the bottom to get out of the way? Of course not—it would cost precious seconds. Before the guy at the bottom had cleared, the guy at the top would come zipping down the pole and land on top of him with the undesired effect of the whole company going out of service due to injuries. To avoid these issues, modern firehouses are all on one floor and the fire pole is now obsolete.

At some point, the guys at our house figured that the safest route to the apparatus floor was via the good old-fashioned stairs, and they abandoned the fire poles altogether. Maybe a few seconds lost, but all bodies arrived at their rigs in one piece. Just as the fire pole was a safety hazard, the stairway had challenges all its own.

Built in an era when horses were still used to pull the fire engine, a spiral staircase had been installed to keep the horses from going up or down the stairs. It was a necessity in the early 1900s, but it was not so functional in modern times.

A beautiful work of art, a narrow wrought-iron spiral stairway connected the basement to the first and seconds floors. If a mistake was made, it was of an unforgiving nature. A trip forward could send you careening headfirst down the steep, metal steps. A slip sideways would set you on a route over the short railing to the basement below.

Due to the high volume of calls, most paramedics chose not to deal with the stairs at all, instead sleeping in the TV room on the first floor with the fleas and rats. I decided to take my chances on the second floor in the bunkroom and with the stairs. I calculated that the most dangerous time to make my way down would be after midnight, when I might be a bit groggy, and formulated what I believed to be a foolproof technique. Maintaining a firm grip on the railing with both hands, if I tripped, I could prevent myself from falling as I corkscrewed around down to the first floor.

At two A.M., I had just sat down on my bed. The cue for the bells to ring was right after I removed one sock, and true to form, one sock off—the overhead blared. "Ambulance 34, take the …." I made my way through the dark bunkroom, dodging occupied beds, the ancient timbers creaking beneath my feet. I headed toward the sliver of light surrounding the door that led to the locker room in which the stairway lay. Round and round I went, with a death grip on the railing. I found myself blinking in darkness, momentarily confused as to where I had been transported until I realized I had taken one too many turns and ended up in the basement.

Everyone spent the day in the kitchen or in the TV room on the first floor. During daylight hours, no one ever went upstairs—avoiding the dreaded staircase. After hours of blaring sirens boring into my brain;

crowded, smelly apartments and uncooperative intoxicated patients whose incontinence assaulted my nose, I would be in a state of sensory overload. Being by myself in a quiet atmosphere, even if it was only for a few minutes, reenergized me. Day or night, whenever we made it back to quarters, I'd tiptoe up the tiny spiral stairs and make my way to the bunkroom. There I would slip into my warm nest. My bed was always made and the dial on my electric blanket cranked to preheat in anticipation of my return.

My partner, Eduardo, thought it was ridiculous for me to make the hike up the death trap staircase only to have to come back down minutes later for another run. He would do the sensible thing and flop down on a flea-infested couch in the TV room. Ed was right; going up and down the stairs was beginning to wear on me, but I couldn't give up my bed. I decided the abandoned fire pole was the answer. During the night, it would be impossible to use the pole, as the trapdoor would have to be left open. With everyone asleep in the dark bunkroom, it would be a safety hazard. However, during the day, it was light out and everyone was downstairs—there was no harm done in leaving it unsecured.

I was a bit nervous about executing a slide, as I had never done it before. It didn't seem like rocket science, and I was pretty athletic. On the other hand, how embarrassing it would be if some disaster occurred while sliding. It would be ammunition for making fun of me for the rest of my career. Case in hand, there was a guy whose nickname was "Sticky Fingers," which he earned while he was candidate. The name followed him all the way to his retirement party. I will leave it up to your imagination as to how he earned this illustrious name.

I had just sat down on my bed at four in the afternoon, peeling off my sock when the bell rang. This was it, my maiden voyage down the pole. I opened one side of the trapdoor and then the other. I took a grip, dangling momentarily, and then wrapped my legs around the pole.

As I hung there, I contemplated my next move. I didn't want to go too fast and risk a crash-landing and ending up in a heap at the bottom of the pole. The grip had to be firm, yet not too firm, or I'd get a friction burn on my hands, I surmised.

I executed a perfectly controlled side, adjusting the grip of my arms and legs as I plummeted downward. I got about three-quarters of the way down and glanced toward the floor, in anticipation of my landing. To my surprise, directly under the pole was a mass of chairs. The guys had been sweeping the apparatus floor and had piled them right at my landing site. I came to a screeching halt.

"Hey, quit messing around. We have a run," Ed said as he made his way to the rig. My "cool" factor had gone down several points and was well into the silly range.

The old firehouse lay empty now. It seems sad after so much life had occupied it for all those years. The day before the move into the new house, I happened to be working in the area. I had recently been promoted to paramedic field chief. Walking through the old place, I felt I should say something significant.

"Farewell old firehouse, good bye old dilapidated building, I had some good times here." However nothing seemed right for the occasion.

The house continues to stand to this day, the same as it had when I first walked through the door some thirty years earlier. With the closing of that old firehouse, something was ending for me and would be lost forever. I realized it wasn't just the firehouse I was pining for. I was losing some part of myself. That young candidate, the new ambulance commander, all of whom I realized were now long gone.

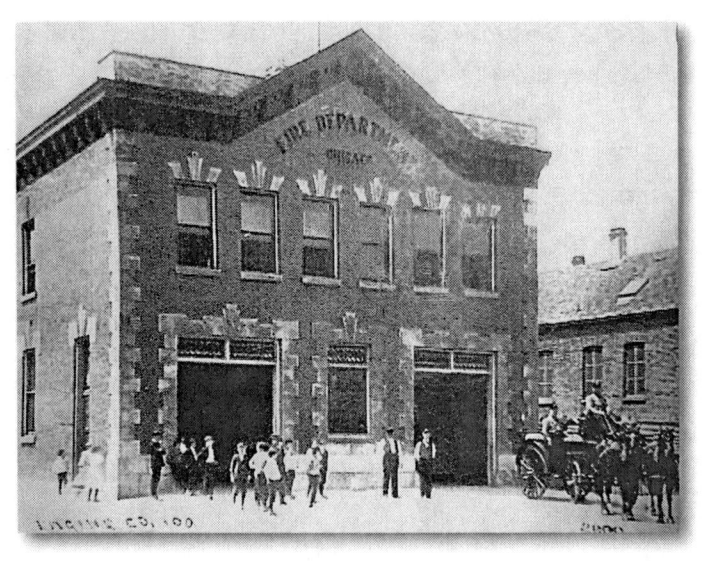

The old firehouse, circa 1907

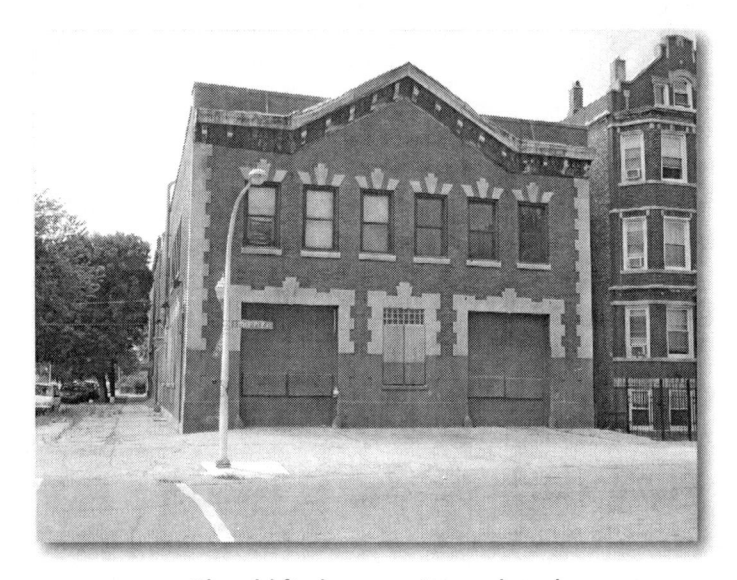

The old firehouse as it stands today

IT'S NOT THE TRAUMA, IT'S THE DRAMA

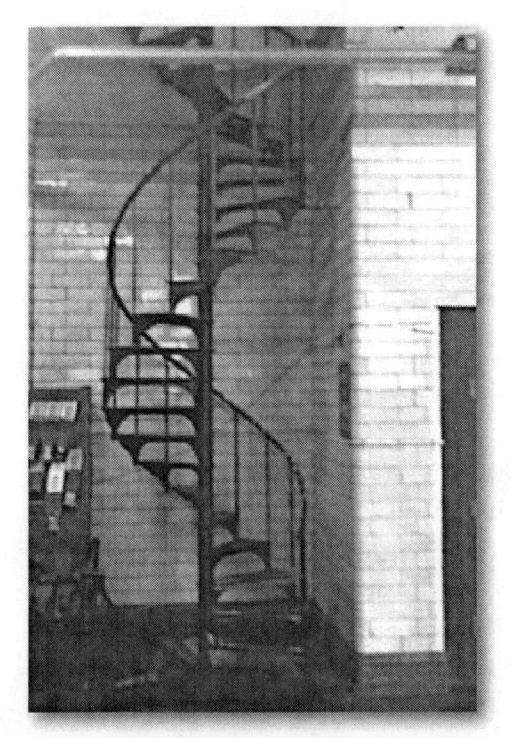

The death trap spiral staircase

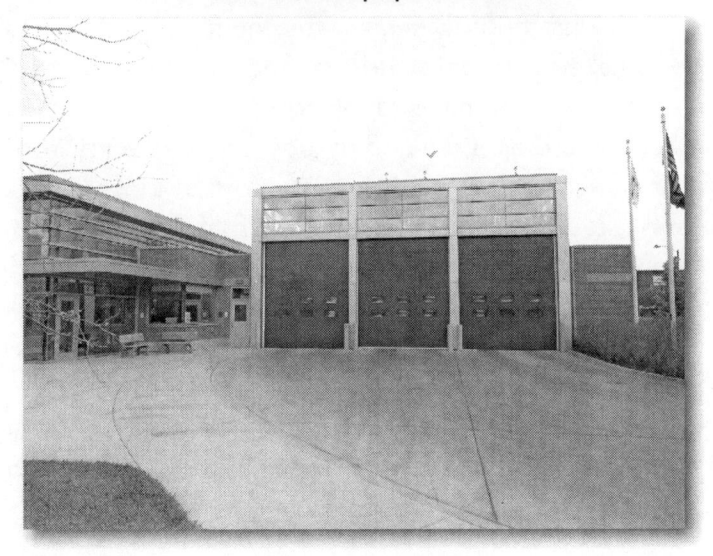

The new firehouse

Truck Guys

When I was a candidate paramedic, I made the unforgivable mistake of confusing an engine for a truck. "Engines have hose, trucks have ladders," I was informed by a disgusted firefighter.

Truck guys are cool; they are the can-do guys on the job. If you need anything done, ask a truck guy. No matter what it is, they will make it happen, and have the tools to prove it. These are the guys on the roof of the fire building, chopping holes to ventilate the interior in order to dissipate heat and smoke so the engine guys can safely enter with their hoses to put water on the fire. Chopping holes in the roof of a building on fire—seriously? Oh, yes. Inside they perform a search and rescue, looking for fire victims. After the fire is out, they take long pointy poles called pike polls and tear apart the walls and ceilings to make sure not a spark remains to rekindle the fire.

Whether you are on a run and request a forced entry into a building, need a patient extricated from an auto that looks like a crushed tin can, or backed the ambulance into a light pole and need the dent taken out of the bumper to save you a mound of paperwork, these are the guys for you. Locked yourself out of your rig? Get a truck guy. A truck officer is the "Jean-Luc Piccard" of the truck company. His mantra is—"Make it so."

Ambulance runs and truck guys can sometimes be like trying to mix oil and water. When they join us on calls, patience or an operation of a delicate nature is occasionally needed when dealing with the public. These characteristics do not necessarily come naturally to the truck guy, as I shall demonstrate in the form of three stories.

• • •

New Year's Eve is the worst day of the year to be on shift. I once did eleven runs after midnight on Ambulance 43; I didn't even know that was possible. Beginning around one in the morning or so, dispatch will traditionally ask, "Are there any ambulances available on the North Side?" This will escalate to, "Are there any ambulances available?" As soon as an ambulance comes up, no matter what their location, they will get the next run. You know dispatch has a stack of calls waiting and are getting desperate. The system is on overload. This is the night when it is not unusual to have response times of fifteen-minutes or more and to go on road trip after road trip.

I was working Ambulance 46 on New Year's Eve 2000. As some of us may recall, this was the night the world as we knew it was supposed to come to an end. Armageddon—computers crashing and mass mayhem in the streets was predicted. Most ambulances had a police escort for protection, an unprecedented move. On Ambulance 46, we had received a roll of tape for our personal protection. We were told to crisscross this clear plastic tape across our windshield in case someone or some thing smashed it. Thanks a lot.

At six A.M., we were running on no sleep. Being up for almost twenty-four hours straight is a feeling that is difficult to describe. What it's not is, "Gosh, I'm tired," it's not even, "Boy, I'm really tired." Gravity is weighing heavily on you. Every molecule in your body hurts, and they're collectively whispering a silent plea, "What are you doing to us? Stop this madness." It's abuse of the body on a cellular level.

We got a call for a psych patient. Psych patients are my personal specialty. I seem to have a calming effect on them, as they innately know they are among one of their own. When I look psych patients in the eye and try to engage them, I can immediately tell if I will have success or not. Their thought process may be completely dysfunctional, but most of the time, some part of them is with me. However, there are the rare occasions when I can't engage on any level and the situation may become volatile. This type of psychotic episode is very dangerous for first responders and needs to be recognized immediately, or someone is likely to get hurt. Sleep deprivation was eating away at my normally compassionate soul as the hours left in my shift slowly ticked down.

Truck 34 was our ambulance assist company. We pulled up to the scene together. The guys exited the rig. Having as bad a night as we were, they looked terrible. Dark circles under glassy eyes were set against pale gray skin. Their hair was in disarray, sticking up at awkward angles. I probably wouldn't have noticed if it was only one or two guys that had looked like that, but they all looked the same. It was comical, not that I was in the greatest condition myself.

We entered a basement apartment to find a twenty-five-year-old male and his girlfriend, who had made the call. She said he had been drinking and smoking crack all night. He had a history of schizophrenia and had threatened to kill himself. I asked him how he was doing. He called me some choice names, not engaging. He just ranted in an incoherent manner.

This was not going to be good, and I did not have the energy to go the extra mile, not that it would have necessarily made any difference.

"Take one of the guys with you and get the stretcher and restraints," I quietly relayed to my partner. The stretcher rolled in which set the patient off again. He stated he wasn't going anywhere and that we couldn't force him to, and then he spewed a stream of profanities. Fortunately, he was all talk and not a lot of action. Without much effort, we were able to maneuver him onto the stretcher and restrain him with the help of five firefighters. Trussed up like a Thanksgiving turkey, we wheeled him outside toward the ambulance. In the crisp winter air, a glimmer of daylight was making its way over the horizon.

As we pulled the stretcher toward the ambulance, he spewed, "Fuck you, I'll kill y—" and then his words were suddenly cut off. I stopped and spun around to see what had caused this unexpected reprieve.

"You better shut up, these are my friends," the truck lieutenant croaked. His reddened face was twisted in anguish as his knee leaned heavily on the patient's throat.

This action had the immediate effect of causing our ward to have a rational thought, which I can assume was, "I best shut up." Eyeballs popping, his mouth snapped shut.

Our Standard Operating Procedure manual does not contain this particular maneuver. Right or wrong, after this nightmare of a shift, it seemed perfect. As soon as the patient settled down, the lieutenant released him, unharmed. He knew he had been beaten, and did not utter a word out of turn for the rest of the ride to the hospital.

All medics lose it at some point in their career. It is due to the stress of dealing with the public, who often call for non-emergencies. I would also venture to guess that some eighty percent of our runs are either drug or alcohol related and a huge percentage also have a psych history. Eventually, something has to give.

The firefighters who join us on ambulance assist runs don't usually lose it as they don't have enough steam built up to blow. They have limited contact with patients and only assist us in the capacity of manpower. I took the lieutenant's actions as not blowing a gasket, but defending us. His knee may have been in the wrong place, but his heart was not.

• • •

The thought process involved in calling 911 can be a mystery. I once had a woman call because she wanted us to smell her sandwich that she thought had gone bad. At times, it is difficult to ascertain what event has initiated the call for help.

I was working on Ambulance 34. At five-thirty in the morning, we had a run for a seizure patient; Truck 32 was our assist company. We were in the kitchen of a home where several adults stood about in silence. No one offered any information as to why they had called. The truck guys were standing by quite patiently; it had been a long night for everyone. Their six-thirty relief was close at hand as I began my inquiry.

"Who called 911?"

"Oh, I did," said a young woman. She then fell silent.

"Who did you call for?"

"My father." Silence again. Extracting information from this woman was going to be frustratingly slow.

"What's the matter with him?"

"He's foaming at the mouth." Now we were getting somewhere.

"Well, where is he?"

"In the bathroom."

"Where is the bathroom?"

"Oh, it's right there"—she pointed to a door next to us—"but he won't come out." I knocked with no response. Then I tried the knob. The door was locked. As I turned to speak to the woman once again, one of the truck guys took ahold of either side of door, and ripped it right off its hinges, like it was a scenery prop, and gently leaned it against the wall.

Standing in the bathroom was a man who had been brushing his teeth, minty foam flowed from his mouth. He stood motionless, with the brush still inserted, and a look of amazement on his face as he turned toward us in disbelief. He wasn't the only one.

I never knew why they had called to 911. It may sound surprising, but I didn't care. People do the strangest things that just don't make sense. In instances when we do need to ask the "why" question, the answer can be quite unbelievable and can leave us wishing we had never asked at all. After twenty-five years on the job, it was really hard to surprise me—or so I thought.

• • •

We had a call for a twelve-year-old male; the run was dispatched as an "injured victim." A young boy lay on his bed with the end of a seven-foot metal curtain rod sticking out of his anus. I'd never seen a curtain rod that long—it went all the way across the room from where he lay on his side on the bed. It was impossible to get him out of the door, much less into the ambulance like that. A delicate situation, as you might imagine. Wow, I've never seen that before, I thought.

I quietly spoke with his mother outside the room as my partner checked his vital signs. "How did this happen?"

"Oh, I'm so embarrassed, but I didn't know what else to do. I tried to get it out, but it's stuck, and he was yelling so loudly. He said he was constipated and was trying to get the poop out." It was an odd story, but mom seemed sincere. There did not seem to be any reason to believe foul play was involved. I took a peek. It was in there all right. I gently tugged, the patient yelped. It was snagged on the fragile tissue.

"Ambulance 34 to dispatch, we need a truck company for assistance."

"The only way we can get him out of here is to cut the rod," I explained to the truck officer. He immediately sent someone down to his rig to get their bolt cutter.

A lone firefighter was dispatched into the room with the cutters in hand; I'm sure the truck officer had sent in the low man in seniority. It wasn't as if any of them would have volunteered to do this. The other truck guys had vanished. It was a rare occasion that his company would abandon him. After a moment of consultation, we decided where to make the cut. However, every time the bolt cutter was placed around the rod, the rod moved a bit causing the kid to scream. Well, we all felt his pain, but it had to be done.

I was losing the truck guy. With each scream, he became more hesitant to cut, pulling the bolt cutters away faster each time.

"You're doing it now, cut, go!" Cutter placed around rod, kid screaming.

"Cut, cut!" I urged as every molecule in his body told him to pull the cutters away. With all his strength, he snipped. The rod easily fell away. We were then able to get the boy out of the room and placed him on his side on the stretcher. I would venture to say that that firefighter would have rather been on the roof of a burning building risking his life than cutting that rod.

You've Got My Eye

My husband's golf cart punched him. Dan had bent over to pick something up off of the floor in our dark garage when the handle of the cart bopped him right in the eye. He made out better than the cart, which ended up being launched across the garage, hitting the wall, and coming to rest in a mangled heap. Dan's eye was red, swollen, and angry. He had scratched his cornea, a very painful and unpleasant injury. Thankfully, he would recover.

My next shift, I was on Ambulance 7, which is located at Belmont and Cicero. I was working with Russ Struts, a laid-back, hardworking guy. It was a hot summer day, so we stopped at a convenience store to get something to drink. At the checkout counter, it caught my attention. Being the thoughtful and dutiful wife that I am, I bought my husband a new eye. It was not just any plastic eye; it was pretty realistic. The eyeball floated inside a clear plastic sphere filled with fluid. It spun round and round; it was also fun to play with. I would present it to Dan the next day, I decided. He would think it was funny—really.

Back at the firehouse, Russ and I rolled the eye back and forth. It glided smoothly and silently across the kitchen table, eyeball slowly spinning and surveying its new home.

"Eh, I like dat eye." said Enzo Morelli, better known as "Cement Head." Enzo looked like a big block of cement, square and stocky with a military-style flattop that had gone all silvery gray. He had taken a fancy to the eye.

Enzo was old-school Italian and spoke the language fluently. He was the driver of Truck 58, and had a cement business on the side. His favorite pastimes at the firehouse were talking cement, loudly fielding phone calls from clients, and sporting his briefcase. He let it be known that it was a very lucrative business. The flip side was that he was about the cheapest guy you could ever meet.

Enzo's hand came down on the eye in mid-slide. He snatched it up and dropped it in his briefcase before snapping the locks shut. "It can keep an eye on tings in my briefcase," he said as he marched out of the kitchen, briefcase in tow.

"Ambulance 7, take the person down from the unknown cause at Belmont and Central." We made for the rig and I lit it up.

"Did Enzo just steal my eye?" I asked Russ as I wrenched the ambulance into gear heading west on Belmont.

"I don't know. Maybe he'll offer to pay for it."

"Enzo pay for it? That's not going to happen, I can't believe he stole my eye!"

"Peg Leg Bob," one of our regulars, was passed out in his usual spot, right in the middle of the sidewalk. We hefted him onto the stretcher, kicking aside an empty bottle of cheap wine, and checked his vitals signs and blood sugar en route to Our Lady of the Resurrection Hospital.

"Wasn't Peg Leg just here this morning?" asked the nurse as we slid him onto the gurney in his usual room.

"Yes, we brought him in first thing. He must have headed straight to the liquor store after he was released." Russ replied.

"If he had just offered to pay for the eye, I would let him have it, but he just took it," I said.

Russ stared at me blankly. I tried to convince myself to let it go. It was only a plastic eye that cost a dollar. I could get another. I was on Ambulance 7 with a busy shift ahead of me. It was, after all, Enzo—a good-hearted guy, but so cheap! The eye to "keep an eye on things in his briefcase." Cute, very funny…but he took my eye!

As Russ finished up the run report at the hospital, I knew without a doubt that I was not going to let it go. Something was going to happen, although I didn't quite know what. Whatever it was, it was going to be good.

"What if we call him?"

"Call who?"

"Call Enzo on the phone and say something using a disguised voice."

Russ, being the good sport that he was, was up for anything, bless his soul.

"How about I say, 'Pay for the eye or die,' and then hang up," he said.

"Oh, that's perfect!"

Russ pulled some crazy voice out of, I don't know where, said his line and gently put the receiver down. We caught a couple of more runs on the air. Every time we got to the hospital, Russ called the firehouse, asked for Enzo, and said, "Pay for the eye or die," and hung up.

Things quieted down and we were on the return to our quarters. Obviously we would be suspect, so I hatched a plan to throw Enzo off. When we got back, he was reading the paper in the kitchen. He briefly lowered it, taking a long hard look at us. Russ immediately snuck into the pay phone in the TV room and called Enzo on the front phone as I sat in the kitchen eating my lunch, which had gone cold hours before.

"Enzo, front phone," blared the overhead.

Enzo picked up the phone and seconds later he slammed it down, "Who the fuck is that?" he bellowed. Sitting down at the kitchen table, he stared straight ahead, looking angry and perplexed. His dark eyes tracked me as I walked to the sink to rinse my dish just as Russ walked in to grab his plate. Oh, we got him. He had no idea what was going on.

"Ambulance 7, take the person down from the unknown cause, 4826 West Byron in the alley." We woke up "Baby Face," another one of our regulars, who was happily snoozing, or rather sizzling on the blacktop next to a Dumpster in the alley. We heaved him onto the stretcher and half-empty bottle of vodka fell out of his pocket and shattered on the ground.

"You would think he would find a more comfy place to sleep it off. Why can't he go into a park under a nice bush where no one would see him," I remarked.

Our Lady of the Resurrection Hospital, or OLR, would not be happy to see Baby Face. He would take up a much-needed room for G-d knows how many hours before he was sober enough to be released, just to head back to the liquor store.

Peg Leg Bob and Baby Face were just a few of our homeless regulars. They referred to each other by their street names, which we eventually picked up on. To be politically correct, I liked to call them our "residentially challenged urban pioneers." This is huge problem throughout the city. Intoxicated homeless people filling up much-needed emergency department beds, sleeping it off, and then sent on their way just to show up again, usually via ambulance.

Russ and I were in conference in the police/paramedic room at OLR. Enzo was on my mind. What to do now? I needed to put the icing on the cake. It had to be something big.

"Enough with the pay for the eye or die. We need to do something else. Any ideas?" I said. After a few minutes, it came to me. This was going to be outstanding!

"What if you say, 'I give you the evil eye,' in Italian?" It would totally throw him off. Obviously, Russ could not possibly know Italian, plus we had both been in the firehouse when he had received his last call.

I phoned my father-in-law, Gino. He was born in Italy and was fluent in Italian.

I explained that I needed to know how to say, "I give you the evil eye" in Italian.

"Why do you want to know this?" he asked.

"Oh, it's just for a joke," I said before briefly explaining the situation to Gino.

"Where in Italy is this guy from?"

"Sicily."

"No, no, no, you can't say that to him. Sicilians take this very seriously."

Somehow I was able to convince Gino to tell me. I had him repeat it slowly several times. I wrote it down, spelling it out phonetically, and handed it to Russ.

"I can't do this, I can hardly speak English," he said. From the corner of the room emerged a Chicago police officer who had been quietly reading a book. He was working security at the hospital; I had barely noticed him. He had overhead the whole conversation.

"I'll do it. What's the guy's name?"

"Enzo."

He dialed the firehouse number. "Close the door," he requested.

"You've got my fuckin' eye. Give me my fuckin' eye!" He yelled at the top of his voice into the receiver. "*Lo ti do il malocchio!*"

He then slammed the phone down, looking quite proud of himself. I was in stitches; Russ was in absolute shock. He had done it with such gusto, and the Italian accent had sounded perfect. After I stopped laughing, wiping the tears from my eyes, I asked.

"Are you Italian?"

"No, Irish."

"Let's get back and see how Enzo is."

We found him in the TV room staring at the set—it was off. The rest of the night flew by with our usual six runs after midnight. I got about an hour of sleep and headed downstairs from the bunkroom at seven A.M. Enzo was already in the kitchen.

The truck had not gone out all night, but he looked worse than I did. Enzo had dark circles under his eyes, and his hair was standing up at crazy angles, in a spiky mess. He looked as if he had been tossing and turning the whole night. With his hands shoved deep in his pockets, he approached me.

"Eh, dat eye, ya know dat eye?"

"Eye, what eye?" I said innocently.
"De eye, to keep an eye on tings in my briefcase."
"Oh yeah, that eye. What about it?"
"Did I ever pay you? How much was it?"
"It was about a dollar."

Fishing around in his pockets, he pulled out a twenty and thrust it toward me. I actually felt kind of bad for him.

"Dat's all I have."
"Don't worry about it. You can get me next time."
"Eh, someone keeps calling me about dat eye, and you know, he speaks pretty good Italian too."

Only a Cut, Please

DID YOU KNOW that the simple act of getting a hair cut could spiral off into some insanely bizarre event? These encounters only occur in an alternate universe known as 911 calls, which is populated by beings that are not like you or me. They either overreact to uneventful incidents, or have little or no reaction to horrific events. Join me for a moment as we step into this peculiar world.

"Ambulance 44, take the shooting at 1625 North Western." As we cruised north on Western Avenue, flashing blue-and-white lights were visible in the distance. Police vehicles had already blocked off the street to civilian traffic. We weaved our way around CPD cars to the front of the building. I grabbed the jump bag and my partner grabbed the stair chair.

We entered a small storefront hair salon. On the ground next to the barber chair, was a woman lying in a pool of blood with a gunshot wound to the side of her head. Brain matter was visible. She was not breathing, and she had no pulse. She was a DOA for sure. Only a couple of feet away on the other side of the room was an adult male lying on his back with a single gunshot wound between his eyes. He was another traumatic arrest/DOA.

I spoke with the police sergeant, "This is going to be a crime scene. They are both DOA. Nothing we can do here."

"OK, sounds good."

"What happened?" I inquired.

"We're interviewing the witness now," he said, pointing in the direction of a guy with half a haircut and still wearing a smock. The witness seemed more pissed off than anything else. I settled in for a moment, taking in the story...

"OK, I'll tell you one more time. I had a one-thirty appointment for a cut. It was just Juanita and me in the store. At about one forty-five, I could see in the mirror that a guy was walking up behind her. He didn't say anything, but it seemed like Juanita recognized him. She started to turn around and that's when he shot her in the head. Then he shot himself between the eyes and fell backward. It was all over in a couple of seconds. That's it! Now, you tell me who is going to fix my hair?"

We finished up our paperwork and informed dispatch it was a crime scene that would be handled by the police. We were back in service. A few minutes later, we got another call.

"Ambulance 44, take the accident at Lake and California." We cruised up to a two-car motor vehicle mishap. I went over to the first car, which had been rear-ended by a second auto and peered inside. Two adult males in their twenties were moaning, each had his seat belt on, and no airbags had been deployed. I approached the open window.

"Hey are you guys OK?" They continued to moan. Not seeing any trauma to either one of them, I asked, "What's the matter—what hurts?" One guy insisted he couldn't move at all, and the other said he had chest pain and couldn't breathe. He seemed to be in no obvious distress. I walked around to the back of the vehicle. There was zero damage. "OK, we'll get you out of there in a few minutes," I said to them.

A quick walk surveying the second vehicle revealed minimal damage to the front end—barely a scratch. "Hey, how ya doing?" I asked the couple in the front seat. The female driver insisted her neck and back hurt, as did the adult male in the front passenger seat. A third occupant had already exited the car and was on his cell phone. His complaint was arm pain. No injuries were visible, and yes, it was the arm with which he was holding the cell phone that he had complained about.

"Do you want to go to the hospital?"

"Yes," they all answered in unison.

"Ambulance 44 to dispatch, we need three more ambulances for a total of four."

During a multi-victim response, of the upmost importance, is gaining an accurate count of how many patients you have and to evaluate the severity of their injuries in order to call for the appropriate number of ambulances. The call could have easily been handled with two more ambulances. In cases of minor injuries, we can transport more than one patient per ambulance. However, two of our victims were insisting that they were severely injured and needed separate ambulances. Good thing there were only five patients, two of whom could be transported together, I thought. If we had any more victims I would have needed an EMS Plan 1, which is a complement of six ambulances, plus a bunch of fire companies for purposes of manpower assistance. That would have been such a waste of resources for this silliness, I thought.

"Hey, over here. Over here!" A man was frantically waving from the sidewalk. He was standing in front of a barbershop and holding his neck. My partner was walking toward the rig to grab some cervical collars to begin treatment.

"I'll go see what this guy wants," I said as I followed him inside a store that looked as if it had not changed since the 1950s. A man was laying next to the barber chair on the floor. "My leg, my leg!" he wailed.

"What happened?" I asked my guide.

"Well, I was giving Mr. Green his usual cut, when we heard a crash outside. He spun around in the chair to see what happened and fell out the chair onto the floor, and I turned my head so fast that I wrenched my neck."

"Do you want to go to the hospital?" I asked.

"Yes."

"Ambulance 44 to dispatch, give me an EMS Plan 1."

Naked Man

"**W**HAT'S WITH ALL the naked people?" I asked my partner Mike after I had been on the job for a few months. "They know we are coming, why don't they put something on? And why do so many people die naked?"

"It's because they came into this world in their birthday suits, so that is how they must go out."

"You put a lot of thought into that, didn't you?"

"Yes, very deep and introspective, is it not?" Mike said sarcastically.

The most important piece of equipment on the job is the blanket. I cannot even relate to you the number of times I've walked into a home with five firefighters in tow and found that the patient was nude, topless, or in their undies. I'm not talking swimsuit models here. I'm talking about grown men and women of every size and shape, the young and even the very old. This nudeness does not remotely correlate to the injury or illness at hand. It would actually make some sense, if, for instance, you had itchy hives all over your body and had your shirt or pants off, but those are the people who have three layers of clothes on. It is the guy sitting completely naked on the couch, his beer belly thankfully covering his prized possession, who is complaining of chest pain. Or, the topless, thirty-five year old, three hundred pound woman who called because she thinks her blood sugar is high.

They called 911; they must have known we were coming, did they not? Yet when we arrive, yes, they are expecting us. And yes, they are in a severe state of undress. No, they could not care less and they act as if it is perfectly normal to be unclothed and opening their door to seven strangers. What is this phenomenon? I have no idea, even after over thirty years on the job. I decided very quickly, as I did with many things, to not even attempt to figure out why people do the strange things they do. I just covered them with a blanket, treated them and moved on. Speaking of moving on, I once had to move on very quickly when I had an unexpected encounter with one such character.

My regular partner, Ben, had made a trade with Ray Kowalski. I was working with him for the twenty-four-hour shift. I recognized the name, but I didn't really know him. We had never worked together. Working with someone new is always an adventure. Everyone has their own quirks and ways of doing things. Somehow you have to mesh with this perfect stranger, figuring each other out as you move through your shift. Most of the time it works, but sometimes it does not.

"Ambulance 46, take the overdose at 5644 North Kedzie, floor three." It was about midnight on a cool April evening. I rolled the rig up to the curb in front of a large three-story apartment complex located in the Ravenswood neighborhood. Ray grabbed the jump bag as I yanked the stair chair out of the side compartment. After making our way up the sidewalk to the outside door of the building, we entered a large vestibule loaded with small metal mailboxes. It was a big building with two doors, one leading to a stairwell on the north side of the building and another door that led to a set of stairs for the apartments on the south side of the building.

"Ambulance 46 to dispatch, is the apartment on the north or south side of the building?" Ray inquired using his portable radio.

"North side, Ambulance 46." Ray wrenched open the north side door and we began our ascent.

We rounded the second floor stairwell. Hearing footsteps, we both stopped and looked up. I saw a pair of hairy legs coming down from the third floor. As the patient descended to the second floor landing, it was clear this individual was naked. Not in the least bit surprised (it's really hard to surprise CFD paramedics), Ray turned around, figuring naked man would follow him down the stairs. This, however, was not to be. Naked man grabbed him by the neck and put him in a chokehold.

I always wondered, never having been a violent person myself, could I hurt someone if I really needed to? I had been on the job for over fifteen years at the time, and had many an occasion in which I needed to restrain a violent patient. I have absolutely no problem jumping in, holding someone down and trussing them up like a Thanksgiving turkey so they cannot hurt themselves or others. But, I've done it in conjunction with my partner, or sometimes with firefighters or police—never by myself.

A berserk naked man was choking Ray. Could I hurt someone if I really need to? Yes I could.

Without a second thought, I had the stair chair in a backswing and was ready to thrust it forward with enough force to knock out a few of naked man's teeth and possibly annihilate his face, when Ray said, "Don't hit him. He doesn't really have me." With that, Ray pulled naked man's arm off from around his neck and proceeded to run down the stairs past me as naked man began to kick him. Not wishing to accost naked man on my own, I had no choice but to turn and run after Ray with naked man in pursuit, three-stooges style. Ray carried the bag, I carried the stair chair, and naked man carried nothing but his intent to do us harm.

At the bottom of the stairs, Ray faced the first obstacle that could slow him down—the door into the vestibule. Not wanting to miss a stride, he dropped the jump bag as he pulled open the door and dashed out. I, on the other hand, had not only the door to deal with, but I also had to deal with the jump bag, which was on the ground directly in front of the door and blocking my exit. I flung the stair chair under my arm, grabbed the bag and wrenched open the door with the other hand.

I know, I know. Why didn't I just dump the stair chair, which would have slowed down naked man and kicked the bag to the side? Do you have any idea of the paperwork involved in lost, damaged or stolen equipment? Piles of paperwork and probably disciplinary action would have followed.

Considering the load I was carrying, Ray was not far ahead of me; he was just outside the front entrance when I heard him call for a 10-1 on the portable radio. A 10-1 is a police code used for "police officer in danger." It means, I need help, and I need it now.

When a paramedic relates this code to dispatch, it's the equivalent of calling out the cavalry. The ambulance was in sight, but naked man was gaining on me. I could hear his naked little feet slapping on the ground close behind me. I had to get to the ambulance, open the door and get in, all without him catching me. It was not possible; plus, I was still hauling all the equipment. To hell with the bloody equipment. I dumped the bag and stair chair at the side of the rig in the street, ran around to the driver's side door, ripped it open, and jumped in. But where the heck was Ray? I had expected him to be in the passenger seat by then, but it was empty. I wanted to lock the doors, but couldn't. I didn't know where he was.

Ray suddenly dashed past my side window and around the front of the ambulance with naked man close at his heels. I rolled down my window.

"Get in!" I yelled. On his next lap around the ambulance, Ray jumped in.

I auto-locked the doors and went to put it in gear with the intent of flooring it.

"Just stay here. It's not like he has a weapon and can hurt us," Ray said.

Reminiscent of old horror movies, naked man appeared at my window with his face not an inch away from it. He stared at me for half a second and then raised his fist with the clear intent of smashing the window in. I peeled out, leaving ambulance rubber all over the road.

I stopped the rig about a block and a half away and pulled over to check in the rearview mirror for the nudie guy's location. He was in the middle of the street. Traffic had stopped. Naked man had his hands on the hood of a car and was attempting to push it. Having no luck, he then lay down in the middle of the street on his back, spread-eagle. Now remember, this is Chicago. We have some of the worst traffic jams in the country. People soon tired of naked man's antics and simply began driving around him. Sirens wailed, and police cars screeched to a halt. Naked man made a beeline for the apartment building running full out—not a pretty sight.

"Ambulance 46 to dispatch."

"46 go."

"We are in service returning. Police are going to handle."

"Message received 46." The police had cuffed and shackled up our man and hauled him off to Swedish Covenant Hospital. I barely spoke a word to Ray the rest of the shift. He made no apologies for his behavior, which had seriously endangered my health and safety. Ray had done the opposite of everything any partner I had ever worked with would have done given the situation. It's never every man for himself. No matter what arises, we are in it together and tackle whatever comes as a unit.

Our next call brought us to Swedish Covenant Hospital. I asked one of the nurses if she could check on naked man's condition. She said he had been admitted to the psychiatric ward with a "rule out drug overdose" diagnosis. They were still awaiting drug-screening results.

Due to my intimate knowledge of human nature, I believe I can extrapolate the events that occurred in naked man's apartment prior to our arrival:

IT'S NOT THE TRAUMA, IT'S THE DRAMA

2300 hours: "I'll be over in five minutes; have the cash ready," said naked man's drug dealer.
2345 hours: "Knock, knock!"
Naked man, fully clothed opens the door.
"I thought you said five minutes. It's been forty-five minutes." Drug dealer guy doesn't really care that he is late. Empathy and punctuality are not his strong points.

Our clothed naked man pays for his goods and the drug dealer leaves. He lights up a joint soaked in PCP and inhales deeply. The room spins; naked man knows he is loosing his grip on reality.

2355 hours: "Man, this is too strong," he thinks, before making his last rational decision for some time.
2357 hours: He picks up the phone and dials. "Hello 911?"
"This is 911, what is your emergency?"
"Please send an ambulance right away.
I smoked some PCP and am really freaking out."
2358 hours: "Sir, the ambulance is on its way. Wait until you see them pull up in front and then remove all of your clothes."

Oh, Shit

"AMBULANCE 46, ENGINE 79, person unconscious not breathing at 6154 North Ponchartrain," the overhead blared.

"Poncha what?" Clayton mumbled.

This was about par for the course since Clayton Jackson had mysteriously arrived via the last transfer order. Clayton lived and had spent most of his career on the South Side of Chicago. He was blissfully ignorant of our complicated North Side area, and apparently wanted it to remain that way. He relied solely on me to safely guide us to the correct location. I found this to be flattering, yet at the same time, alarming.

"What's going to happen when I'm on furlough?" I asked him as he dozed off in a La-Z-Boy chair with a pile of area maps in his lap that I had thrust at him. I had learned my lesson the hard way by getting terribly lost at a most inconvenient time.

When disaster struck, I was working with Wally Piatkiewicz. The year was 1998—pre-GPS. Wally was somewhat familiar with the area, but he was only working with me for the shift. It was my assignment; therefore, he was counting on me to know my area. We had been returning from Resurrection Hospital when we got the call.

"Ambulance 46, Still and Box alarm at 6831 North Nokomis." A Still and Box is not only a fire, but a pretty big one.

"Know where that is?" Wally asked.

"I think so." I was not so sure.

IT'S NOT THE TRAUMA, IT'S THE DRAMA

The Wildwood and Sauganash neighborhoods are areas like no others in Chicago. The streets are not set out in a sensible, systematic grid-like pattern as is most of the rest of the city. It is as if the city planner went off his meds and started hallucinating—or maybe magic mushrooms were involved. Angle streets intersect angle streets. Streets begin and abruptly end a block later, only to be continued miles away not only once, but in several instances twice. The same street could be at separate locations miles apart.

The street names are also quite interesting—Dowagiac, Minnehaha, Sioux, Hiawatha, etc., indicate the area's Native American roots. Surely the white man had stripped this land away from the Native Americans. If revenge could be had, as it should have been, it was had in the layout of these streets, as many a white man has taken a wrong turn in that blasted neighborhood.

A fire in this upscale area is highly unusual. To complicate matters, it is home to most of the firefighters and paramedics who live on the North Side of Chicago. It's not a great time to be meandering about, when your off-duty colleagues at home are sure to spot the smoke and show up at the fire scene in droves.

With all this laying heavily on my mind, we took another turn for the worse. I realized I did not know where this street was after several failed attempts to find it. Wally jumped in as I was out of ideas.

"Turn here. I think it's in this neighborhood in the woods off of Devon and Central."

It wasn't. Shit, shit, shit, I thought, feeling the heat rise in my face. I was letting Wally down. The whole department was probably on the scene wondering where we were. What if there were injuries? Shit, shit, shit!

"Ambulance 46, what is your location?" dispatch demanded.

"We are on the scene." Out of sheer luck, I had somehow stumbled upon the fire scene. The possible consequences of my incompetence were racing through my mind as we made our embarrassingly late entrance. Disciplinary action could follow, along with a humiliating confession professing my ineptness. Shit, shit, shit!

"What took you so long?" asked our paramedic field chief. Wally, angry beyond words, did not speak.

"Sorry," I said.

"We have a guy who set his house on fire and covered himself in feces. He needs to get a psych evaluation."

By the time we arrived, the fire had been extinguished. A slightly singed and smoldering man was standing on the front porch of his home. His naked body was covered in feces, which was smeared with great care from the top of his head down his torso, across both arms, and down and around his legs to the tips of his toes.

"Oh, shit," Wally grumbled.

A Heck of a Party

"**W**HAT IS THE worst thing you have ever seen?" my civilian friends would repeatedly ask me. My friend Esther asked me this once. She cuts hair in an upscale hair salon. To me her job is much scarier than mine; you're messing with someone's hair.

Can you imagine screwing up and having to carry the burden every day of knowing someone is looking in the mirror and silently cursing you? Would you want to be responsible for someone's bad hair day for six weeks? It's all too much for me. You have to be tough as nails to be in that business, so I figured she could take it.

I relayed a somewhat gruesome call I had had recently, which wasn't even the worst thing I had ever seen. Her response was, "Don't ever tell me anything again," as she gave me a strange sideways glance as if I had just committed some heinous crime.

After that disastrous encounter, I used the technique of bait and switch, quickly changing the subject before the perpetrator of the question could realize I was telling them a story filled with life, hope, and humor instead of disemboweled bodies. This is the story I would tell:

I was working with my regular partner, Ben. This was prior to his leaving me to go to greener pastures on an ambulance in the Norwood Park neighborhood.

"You know, Ambulance 39 does the exact same number of runs that we do, except they are much busier at night," I told Ben for the umpteenth time, trying to get him to stay.

Your partner leaving is a terrifying event. A good partnership is a relationship like no other, and you don't know who you will get when they leave. Once they have left, it's an arranged marriage with the outcome determined by who is the most senior person who bid on the assignment.

You see each other at your absolute best and worst. For example: it's your sixth run after midnight, and it's for someone who called 911 because he had a nightmare that he would like to relay to you in intimate detail at five in the morning, as if we had nothing better to do. Your partner is about to lose it, when you calmly step in, because you know without words being exchanged, that he needs you to deal with this person as his patience meter is on empty. At your best, you work without speaking, both on the same page, using techniques you have learned to actually save someone's life.

"Ambulance 46, take the chest pain victim at 3935 West Devon Avenue."

"That's Monastero's, isn't it?" Ben asked. Monastero's is a fixture in the Peterson Park neighborhood. It's a restaurant and banquet hall. It's also a popular place for wedding receptions.

As we pulled up, a man in a tux waved us into the banquet hall; loud music assaulted our ears as we were quickly guided into the men's bathroom toward our patient.

Sol, a man in his fifties, was sitting on the floor. He was experiencing a sudden onset of severe chest pain, weakness and shortness of breath. In medical terms, he looked like crap. He was pale and had broken out into a cold sweat called diaphoresis.

We generally like to work our patients where they lie, but with music blaring and about twenty-five of his closest relatives jammed into the bathroom, we put Sol on the stair chair and made a quick escape to the ambulance, which was a short distance away.

Sol had no medical history. He had been on the dance floor celebrating his daughter's wedding when his symptoms had begun. Vital signs revealed a hypotensive, tachycardic patient with mild respiratory distress. Oxygen was administered; a heart monitor was applied. When the reading appeared on the monitor screen, Ben and I gave each other "the look." I quickly slipped an IV into his vein. The monitor revealed ventricular tachycardia, a fatal heart rhythm if left untreated.

"Hey, Sol, your heart is beating kind of funny. That's what's causing your chest pain and low blood pressure. We're going to have to zap you with a bit of electricity to get your heart beating correctly," Ben explained.

"I have to tell you, it's going to hurt, so we'll give you something for the pain first. Are you ready?"

"Go for it," Sol replied.

I injected six milligrams of Valium, a sedative and pain killer into his IV. Defibrillator pads were in place, and the heart monitor was set to synch at 100 mega joules. It was going to be combination of polar opposites—a serene and peaceful feeling of relaxation, compliments of the Valium followed by a horrendous dose of electricity coursing through his body. The defibrillator juiced up to 100 mega joules, and zap!

Sol's eyes became as big as dinner plates, his body jolted and then relaxed. Ben and I held our breath, our eyes transfixed on the monitor screen, hoping the V-fib had converted to a normal heart rhythm.

The deadly, jagged, shark-toothed-like heart rhythm had thankfully converted to a normal heart rhythm. The change in Sol's appearance was immediate. His color returned as he loudly announced—"Wow! You guys throw a heck of a party!"

Imagine

I KNOW YOU ARE dying to know and can take it if you are reading this, so here goes nothing. It's the worst thing I have ever seen.

Imagine you are driving north on the Edens Expressway, just south of the Peterson Avenue exit. The expressway takes an eastward zig, then a slight westward zag. It's four-thirty A.M. on a Saturday morning that will soon blossom into a lovely warm June day. However, it is not quite morning yet—it's that in-between time, that time just before sunrise. It's still dark out, but the birds are chirping away. You are a bit tipsy as you were downtown on Rush Street drinking with a couple of buddies. As you come around the zig part of the Edens, you see an ambulance with its lights on parked on the east side shoulder of the expressway.

"Hey, pull over. Let's see what's going on," one of your buddies suggests.

You slowly guide your car off the expressway and stop about a hundred feet south of the ambulance. You and your buddies exit and begin to walk north. Two paramedics are standing over something by the guardrail. They don't notice you at first, as they are talking. You walk closer to see what has their attention.

"Oh my G-d!" You vomit up about $30.00 worth of kamikazes.

• • •

Imagine you are quite intoxicated, having spent the night—well, actually about the last fourteen hours—in the Bim Bom Lounge on Belmont Avenue.

The bar closed at four A.M. and the owner kicked you out. You thought there was time for just one more; he thought not.

It's really hot outside, so you shed your shirt, leaving it in the parking lot as you mount your motorcycle, the engine coughing to life. You head toward home on the Edens Expressway North, feeling freer than you ever have. Unencumbered by helmet or shirt, you sense the power of the bike beneath you. You feel indestructible and surpass one hundred miles per hour as you round the zig in the Edens just south of Peterson Avenue, just before the zag. Suddenly, as if a carpet has been pulled out beneath you, you are sliding. The bike is at a strange angle; there is no traction. You ask yourself, how did this happen? Why am I sliding? Everything is in slow motion, yet you are traveling very quickly. The guardrail is getting closer and closer, then there's a flash of light.

• • •

Imagine you are a paramedic on Ambulance 46 working with one Clayton Jackson. You have had a pretty good day, and thankfully are in a deep slumber in the bunkroom at your quarters located at Peterson and Pulaski Avenues. Imagine you are rudely awakened from your slumber at four-thirty A.M. by a computerized female voice stating, "Ambulance 46, take the motorcycle accident on the Edens Expressway, outbound south of Peterson Avenue." Just in case you did not hear the bazillion-decibel computerized voice, a shrill ringing of the same, if not a higher volume assaults your eardrums.

"Hey Clay, isn't that where the Edens zigs and then zags?"

"Sure it is. I hope this guy didn't zag instead of zig."

"We'll have to get on at Foster and then head north," I said. As we careen down the entrance ramp onto the Edens at Foster, I scan left, Clayton scans to the right. At this hour of the morning, there's no traffic; however, the light is not good. It's that strange other-worldly light that is cast at the intersection between night and day—and those damn birds—what are they chirping about? It's still dark out for G-d's sake!

At first we see nothing at all. Clayton is ready to ask dispatch if they have any more information.

"What's that?" I say, pointing at something lying on the east shoulder of the expressway. We cruise over and step out.

It's a pair of blue jeans perfectly arranged with one leg in it, shoe included with the laces still tied. It's as if someone had lay down to rest and then suddenly gotten up and fled the scene, leaving his pants and one leg behind.

"Where's the rest of him?" Clay asks. We both walk about thirty feet north of the leg along the guardrail and then stop. "Oh, there he is."

"I wonder where the head is?"

We both turn at the same instant to see a bunch of kids vomiting.

"Hey, you wanted to see it," Clayton remarks.

We better cover him up before we get any more gapers." I go to the rig to retrieve two sheets, one for the leg and another for the rest.

• • •

Imagine you are a mom. It's eight-thirty in the morning, and you are driving car pool. Hannah, your oldest at age seven, is in the front seat. Nathaniel, age four, is in the back seat, but he's somehow making Eli, who is Hannah's age, cry.

"Nathaniel, what are you doing?"

"No'ting, Mama."

"He is being mean. He is so mean to me and he hits me." sobs Eli.

"Nathaniel, cut it out please."

Rose, Eli's younger sister who is also four, will be dropped off at preschool with Nathaniel after I drop off Hannah and Eli at kindergarten. Imagine this mom had just gotten home from work that morning, seven-thirty A.M. to be exact. Imagine she had seen the body of what used to be a man mangled beyond recognition a few hours earlier. Should she act any differently? Should she do anything differently than she was doing now, driving car pool and trying to get her four year old to behave? Well, I don't know, but that is how it was.

• • •

The rest of the body was wrapped around the base of the guardrail. It was a mound of flesh at first unrecognizable. Upon further inspection, there were the lungs and the heart. The chest cavity was split open revealing its contents. We couldn't find the head and thought it may have made it's way to a separate location as the leg had. However, it was lying at an unnatural angle, crushed and in the midst of the blob, the other leg was also wrapped up in the mass of flesh. It was as if the body had been shot from a catapult, landed on the upright of the guardrail, spun around several times, and come to rest in a heap. That, gentle reader, is the worst thing I have ever seen.

The Specter

HISTORICALLY, THERE HAVE been true psychopaths on this job. Somehow they endure and become our bosses. The crazier they are, the more likely they are to be promoted; that's the way it goes on the Chicago Fire Department. It is a vicious cycle because these nuts have huge egos that are constantly being fed by people who have to kiss their appointed asses because they are in charge—this being a semi-military organization, you cannot question them.

They do not take a test; they know someone who knows someone. Once launched into the stratosphere of appointed positions, they orbit about for all eternity, occasionally changing titles. They have no intention of retiring because they are immortal due to their allegiance with "the dark lord." Therefore, we can never escape them.

The psychopath strikes terror into the hearts of caring souls because of one, and only one characteristic they all share—they have no empathy, no idea of how another person might feel. That is why they are capable of such damage. They feel nothing but a desire to control. Their priorities are somewhat askew due to a deranged thought process brought on by their subconscious, which puts them, not the sun, at the center of the universe. OK, OK, one of the guys I'm talking about was the fire department inspector. That was one of his many titles.

I had just been promoted to paramedic field chief and was working overtime at 4-5-2. It is located at Damen and Grace, Engine 112's quarters on the northeast side. I had gotten the call to work overtime on my off day and had been sitting at a spot on the South Side. My gear and uniform were miles away. I put together some extra bedding and borrowed the off-going field chief's fire gear. I had an extra uniform at home, except for the little cross tie we had to wear. I hatched a plan to pick one up at a uniform store before I went for my meeting at Field Division North Headquarters when the 0800 bells rang. It was not the regular ring like, yeah, yeah, the cook is collecting money for the food club. This was a serious ring that only occurs when someone important has arrived at the firehouse. It signifies that all members should go to the apparatus floor immediately.

Everyone was lined up next to their rig when the fire department inspector, Chief Brackin, sauntered in to survey the troops. Tall and thin, he stood erect as a pencil. A crown of gray stubble encircled his balding head. He had gleaming black leather boots with a riding crop in hand (just kidding).

Close set hawk-like eyes zoomed in and out like a periscope scanning each member. Turning in my direction, he hit his target as his eyes burned a hole in my neck.

G-d dammit, I thought. I hate this guy. He took his time, strolling toward me for the maximum effect.

"Do you have your tie?"

"Yes, it's in my car."

"Go get it."

I hate this guy!

"Listen, I do have it, but it's at Engine 88's quarters. I got called for overtime and was going to pick one up today." Yes, yes, I know. I should have gone out to the car and not come back, but I was rattled. How can a grown, married woman with two children, a professional of thirty years be made to feel like a ten-year old who is in big trouble? It was ridiculous.

My next workday, I was thankfully working many miles away. That morning before I left for my shift, I had a tiny spat with my husband.

"You look like an idiot with that tie on," he teased.

"I have to wear it."

"The battalion chiefs only wear their ties when they go to district.

"Fine!" I ripped the tie off and stuffed it into my pocket.

I had just stepped in the door of 4-5-6's quarters, which is the paramedic field chief located on the far southeast side in the Pullman neighborhood, when I caught a run for a working fire. Monitoring the radio on the way over, it didn't sound like much. I parked my buggy about a half block away from the fire building and exited, donning my helmet and turnout coat.

I proceeded toward Sector 1, the front of the building. I heard the battalion chief hold everyone up because the fire was out and my services were not needed. As I turned to heading back toward my vehicle, a dark shadow was cast upon me—I felt a cold chill go through my body. I quickly spun around...

The Specter (spek'tor) noun.

1. A ghostly apparition; phantom
2. A haunting or disturbing image

was once again upon me. It was Chief Brackin, the fire department inspector.

"Where is your tie?" I fumbled in my pocket and made several attempts to put the blasted thing on, but it was all wrong, upside down, and backwards. I have no recollection of what he said to me, but The Specter soon dispatched a memo throughout the city.

The memo was sent to my bosses north and south. It specifically mentioned my name, and said I had been found to be out of uniform without my tie not only once, but twice, and how we need to set an example, etc, etc. Anywhere I went, north or south, I was made sport of—"Hey, where's your tie?" First of all, what were the chances of running into this guy on opposite ends of the city? And second of all, I always wear my tie. Really.

A few work days later, I was dispatched to a three-ambulance response for an auto accident. When I arrived, someone who originally had not wanted to go to the hospital changed his mind. I called for another ambulance. It was not a serious injury.

When I got back to quarters, my boss called. He sounded nervous. "Why did you wait so long to call for another ambulance? Why didn't you call for a Plan?"

"A Plan? For what?" An EMS Plan 1 is a compliment of six ambulances along with a bunch of fire companies used for manpower, traffic control, etc., I didn't need anything like that; it was just one patient, nothing serious at all. What was his problem?

"Chief Brackin wants you to write a Form 2 as to why you didn't call for a Plan."

The Specter had changed hats and was now a district chief. He must have been monitoring the radio and heard my transmission. I wrote the blasted Form 2. We have a different chain of command than the firefighters. I made it out to my assistant deputy chief paramedic. The Specter wouldn't even see it, so what was the point? And how had he known it was me, and why should he have cared what I did or didn't do?

My next work day, I had to pick up some paperwork at fire district headquarters. As I passed by the door of one of the offices, I heard, "Do you have that Form 2?" It was him again, The Specter. We don't give our paperwork to the fire side of the administration. EMS and fire are two separate entities that don't mix paperwork. I told him I had given it to my assistant deputy chief paramedic. He insisted he wanted a copy. I told him I didn't have it with me.

A few weeks later, I ran into him at district again and it was the same thing. He wanted a copy of the Form 2. Why did I keep running into this guy? It was as if we were star-crossed characters in some sort of ill-fated Shakespearean tragedy. Looking for direction, I told another boss that Chief Brackin kept hassling me for the Form 2. It was highly unusual. "You don't have to give him anything," I was relieved to hear.

Now this was getting a little funky. There were several ways to look at this situation:

Scenario 1: Brackin is an asshole and everyone knows it. I'm not the only one he is doing this to, so I shouldn't take it personally. Ignore him as much as humanly possible.

Scenario 2: Brackin is an asshole and everyone knows it. However, he has chosen to single me out for some unknown reason.

Scenario 3: Brackin is an asshole and everyone knows it. He is trying to intimidate me because he is a bully, and I am fanning the fire by not reacting. In effect, I'm letting him bully me, which is a sign of weakness. Bullies like that.

I generally have a pretty good understanding of human nature, but I am like a deer in the headlights when it comes to what to do about situations such as this. How to react in a way that this creature can comprehend and get him to leave me alone was eluding me.

I have tried in the past to have a humanoid conversation with types such as him; it's just no good. They are on a different wavelength. It is a waste of time and has absolutely no effect—or has the opposite effect and spurs them on. After much contemplation, I compiled a set of possible solutions:

Solution A: Continue to have as little reaction and interaction as possible. However, that makes me feel like a wimp.

Solution B: Next time an incident occurs, be defiant and use the "f" word a lot.

Solution C: Sit down with him and attempt to have a "heart to heart," explaining my feelings and requesting his thoughts on the matter.

Solution D: Punch him in the breadbasket and hope for the best, which would include knocking the wind out of him and him doubling over in pain.

I liked Solution D the best, as I firmly believed it would have a most desirable outcome even if it involved suspension, a night in jail, and a court appearance. If I were a guy, that's what I'd have done. It would have been a trip to the alley where all would have been settled like gentlemen. But I am a chick—damn these ovaries! Damn this blasted estrogen that whispers to me to turn the other cheek and talk about my feelings. Damn my childhood that did not involve fistfights or brawls. I know I could have done it if I only had some experience at it.

"Take the working fire at 1943 West Lunt." I was working 4-5-2. I was at the south end of my district, on Belmont Avenue when I got the call. It would be a hike. I lit it up and headed north.

Monitoring the fire radio, I could tell the fire was getting out of control. "Emergency, give me a Box," Battalion 9 requested. The fire had escalated from a "Working Fire" to a "Still and Box" alarm. I had two ambulances on the scene already, Ambulance 56 and Ambulance 13. I rolled up and parked it about two blocks away from the fire building. That was as close as I could get with so many fire apparatus on the scene. Ambulance 13 was treating a civilian burn victim and stated via radio that they were assuming triage.

I put on my turnout coat and helmet, grabbed my clipboard and relayed an EMS staging area and tactical channel to dispatch.

Smoke enveloped me as I made my way toward Sector 1. A white coat was just in front of me—it was a fire chief of some sort whom I could barely make out in the thick haze until he unexpectedly whirled about blocking my path—It was The Specter.

"Do you have your bunker pants?"

I hate this guy!

"Yes."

"Go put them on."

If we attempt to look at this from any perspective that might possibly make sense, such as safety perhaps, I cannot believe, as much as I'd like to believe in the innate goodness of people, that The Specter was concerned with my personal safety.

If I were a firefighter who was going into a fire building without bunker pants, that would have been a major problem. However, there was zero possibility that I would be entering the fire building, or, for that matter, getting particularly close to it.

My job is to evaluate and monitor the situation, be it a civilian or member injured and make sure we have enough medical resources, and give a progress report to dispatch.

"I have patients. I need to see what's going on." I firmly, yet calmly relayed to The Specter. "Go put your bunker pants on now!" he bellowed. Keep in mind that this was a Still and Box Alarm in an occupied building that was continuing to evade being extinguished. There was already an injury on the scene and he was worried about my pants?

I trudged back two blocks. I had to remove my helmet, turnout coat, and shoes, struggle into boots, and pull up bunker pants as the fire escalated to a 2-11 alarm. Not only had I had a delay to the scene, due to his confrontation with me, so had The Specter.

We ended up having two civilian transports and one injured firefighter. If The Specter wanted me to wear bunker pants and boots, any other time would have been a more appropriate moment to mention it. It was ridiculous, sure, but I am a reasonable person. Because this is a semi-military organization, sometimes you just have to do what the incident commander says, and take it with a grain of salt.

I sometimes fantasize about punching him, really causing some damage and seeing the surprised look on his pinched face; or having a mature, adult conversation with The Specter. Maybe he's not a bad guy after all. Perhaps we end up being buds and have a good laugh about it all. Most likely, neither of those will ever occur. What I do know with all my heart is that—I hate that guy.

Thinking Outside of the Box

AFTER TWENTY-FIVE YEARS of working on the ambulance, I was promoted to the rank of paramedic field chief. I would oversee eight to ten ambulances, depending on the district in which I was working. It's a middle management job that lies somewhere in that gray area between being one of the guys, and being their boss. It's like a high-wire act. Fall one way and you lose authority because you are too much of a pal to the troops. Fall the other way and you lose respect because you are too dictator-like.

I was at the top of my game on the ambulance; my skills had been honed over many years. There was nothing I hadn't seen or done. It was fun, because no matter what monkey wrench was thrown at me, I could effortlessly turn any situation into child's play. What I loved best was the endless variety of calls; no two were exactly the same. From one minute to the next, you could never predict what was going to happen.

The field chief gig was a whole new ball game. Very little could be translated from my experience on the ambulance. It was like starting over. The job is one-third administrative (I'd rather take a sharp stick to the eye), one-third mandatorily dispatched runs like a multi-ambulance response or a fire, and one-third that could be anything under the sun. It's the anything-under-the-sun runs that I like best.

On my first day as a paramedic field chief, I rolled out of 4-5-1's quarters, which is located in downtown Chicago. As I slid behind the wheel, I made a mental check to make sure I had everything. Portable radio—check. Manpower—check. My route—check. One forest of trees destroyed to create various pieces of BS administrative paperwork—check. I put the buggy it in gear and cruised out of the door on my maiden field chief voyage.

Do you know that feeling you have when you have forgotten something really important, but you can't for the life of you remember what it is? I had that. I went through my mental checklist again. I had everything, but something was missing. It came to me all at once. How about my partner? How about my ambulance? How about I have no idea what I'm doing? Telephone, telegraph, tell a firemen—If I screwed up, it would be all over. Everyone would hear my missteps on the radio—they all talk! I decided to do a mental check-in with myself every hour on the hour. The checklist consisted of:

1. Did you do anything stupid?

I found I had to do a self check-in every half hour instead; an hour was too much time during which I could screw up. I then went to every fifteen minutes and eventually settled on every ten minutes. That seemed to work best. If I could just make it through the first few months and get some runs and experience without doing something idiotic, I think I could do this.

"You're so lucky. Paramedic field chief is the best job on the department," was all I heard for months after my promotion. I never thought that I would make it to that position, yet there I was, a chief. If I was so amazingly lucky, then why did I absolutely hate the job? It was a terrible secret I had to keep. I certainly couldn't tell anyone; they would have sent me for a psych evaluation.

I didn't take to my field chief duties as seamlessly as everyone else seemed to, and instead I pined for the fun and camaraderie of the ambulance. The worst part was that I had to roll alone.

Paramedic. In Greek, *para* means side by side. The only thing by my side was an empty seat. It sucked. If you have a halfway decent partner, you rely on each other for many things, from how to handle a call and treat a patient, to getting to the run, etc. My only partner was my GPS, which was not good company by any means. I did, however, have many a heated exchange with it, especially when it tried to direct me down railroad tracks while I was working on the far southeast side in the Hegewisch neighborhood. And downtown? Forget it, it was completely schizophrenic.

I was working on the West Side at 4-5-4, which is located at Engine 117's quarters, when I caught a run on the air.

"4-5-4, Chicago and Austin." That was it. That was the only crumb of information dispatch offered me—the address, not even an address—it was an intersection.

I could have been dispatched to that location for any numbers of reasons, the underlying cause being that the paramedics, and or firefighters on the scene had a problem that they needed my help with. The details of the situation would only to come to light once I arrived.

It was all good then. I had been a field chief for over five years. It was a fun run, an anything-under-the-sun run, my favorite.

I pulled up to find a CTA bus facing north on Austin Boulevard. Surveying the scene as I pulled up, I saw no damage to the bus. Tower Ladder 14, an advanced life support truck company (a fire company that includes a paramedic and advanced life support equipment), and Ambulance 83, a basic life-support ambulance with two firefighter/EMT's, were on the scene. The lieutenant on the tower ladder filled me in on what had occurred. The bus driver had slammed on the brakes to avoid a bicyclist who had darted in front of him, which had caused injuries to two passengers on the bus. Prior to my arrival, Ambulance 23 had made a hasty getaway for reasons that would soon become apparent. They had already transported a woman who said her elbow hurt to West Suburban Hospital, which was only about four blocks south of our location. One patient remained on the bus.

A large man in a wheelchair was complaining of neck and back pain—he was loudly threatening to sue the fire department and the CTA. The firefighters and EMT's were visibly shaken, as he had threatened to take legal action if his three-hundred-pound electric wheelchair was not transported with him to the hospital. There was no possibility that his chair would fit into the ambulance with him.

The two problems I faced were how to get his chair to the hospital and how to avoid ending up in court. To complicate matters, the patient's blood pressure and blood sugar were sky-high. The guy was going to blow a gasket if we didn't get him medical treatment quickly, although he did seem to enjoy having everyone scurry about nervously at his threatening manner. He was not a nice guy.

The first line of attack was to get him medical attention. I had the basic life- support ambulance convert to an advanced life-support ambulance by having the paramedic and his equipment from the tower ladder truck transferred to it. The patient was then wheeled down the bus ramp toward an awaiting stretcher.

The wheelchair—what to do about that mongo wheelchair? Even if I called for another ambulance to transport just the chair, I didn't think the firefighters could lift it in. The back of the ambulance was just so darn high. If they could get it in, they could then throw the stretcher from the ambulance onto the top of the tower ladder. As the patient glided down the handicap-accessible bus ramp in his chair, raging about the abuse of the handicapped, how much his wheelchair cost, and that we would be seeing him in court—the idea hit me.

The CTA supervisor was at my side with a worried look on his face. I'm sure he was contemplating the pile of paperwork he was going to have to deal with.

"Hey, can you take his chair to the hospital in the bus?" I asked him.

"Sure," he answered, with a huge smile, as he also realized our friend would not have much of a court case now. After transferring our patient onto the stretcher, we rolled the wheelchair right back up the ramp and locked it into place on the bus. I told him that the bus was going to take his wheelchair to the hospital.

"But it's a northbound bus," he complained.

"Not anymore." I said.

With the patient treated and safely tucked into Ambulance 83, they turned south on Austin Boulevard and headed toward West Suburban Hospital with the bus close behind. Motorcade-style, I fell in line next, and the tower ladder picked up the rear.

The bus pulled right up next to the ambulance at the entrance to West Suburban Hospital's Emergency Department. As the patient was being unloaded from the ambulance, the wheelchair careened down the CTA bus ramp directed via its joystick, at the helm was the lieutenant from the tower ladder. He guided the wheelchair right along side the stretcher, like a well choreographed ballet was being performed, as we made our way into the Emergency Department. The chair was parked next to our ward, who had been transferred onto a hospital gurney in a room that had been waiting for him.

Our patient's entire ploy had been foiled; he was silent and sullen, and made a last gruff request that we put the brakes on his wheelchair.

At the hospital, I hung out with the paramedics on Ambulance 23 as they finished up their report. "Nice getaway," I said about their abrupt departure from the scene.

"Yeah, what a piece of work that guy was. What happened to his chair?"

"Oh, it's right next to him—it barely left his sight."

"What?"

After I relayed the story to them, one of the paramedics said, "Now that's thinking outside of the box."

"No," the other guy said. "She made the box."

Read a story from Marjorie Leigh Bomben's next book,
CFD Shorts; More Stories by a Chicago Fire Department Paramedic

The Democratic Committeemen

WE HAD BEEN dating for about three months. He was in love, I was not. When he insisted on introducing me to his mother, I knew it was time to get out. Extricating myself from a relationship as lopsided as this one was going to be a delicate operation. Just as a neurosurgeon maps out his strategy to remove a tumor from the brain with the utmost of care, taking into account every possible detail of what could go wrong, it was in this spirt that I planned my breakup with Mike. Sometimes, no matter how well a plan you have laid, events that you never took into account occur, setting you on a course into uncharted territory.

It was February 1983. Mike and I had met while working on a private ambulance and had just been hired by the Chicago Fire Department—we were in the same class. This was a bad time for a breakup. While in the Fire Academy, I would have to see Mike almost every day for the next three months.

Our time in the Academy prepared us for nothing. It was a bunch of pomp and circumstance, having little to do with the reality of what we were going to face in the field. Puffed up instructors pranced about like peacocks, their extravagant tails in full display. They had not been on the job much longer than I, yet thinking an awful lot of themselves when given a small taste of authority over a class of new candidates.

I learned exactly two things in the Fire Academy that were ever of any use to me. "The Chicago Fire Department is a semi-military organization." This did not sit well with me, as I was repulsed by authority. A true rebel without a cause. I had to maintain the appearance of conforming—snapping to attention and saluting whenever some chief walked by in the hallway or entered our classroom. How repulsive. But it was good, taming the anti-social, nonconformist in me.

"This is a legal document," we were told of the run reports we generated for every patient. Even after I had been on the ambulance for over twenty years, I would evaluate my report form a lawyers point of view—one who was out to get me as we were often caught up in court cases.

I was kind, I was friendly, yet firm in my delivery of the message that it was over. I had ripped the bandaid off in one fell swoop. It was over with Mike, or so I thought. After the breakup, a series of calls and hang-ups ensued. At two in the morning, before he could hang up, I said, "Mike, I know it's you, what's going on?"

"I'm going to kill myself if we don't get back together. I have a bunch of Valium and a syringe. I'm going to do it." I was not familiar with what the procedure was for this particular situation, but what I did know was that he was not going to kill himself. This was some sort of ill conceived strategy to get me back. He couldn't possibly have made himself more unappealing. Kill himself? Oh, OK I'll be right over, and by the way, I really do love you! Honestly—how ridiculous.

The next day, I put in a call to his sister and told her what had transpired. She assured me she would tell her mother so they could both talk to him. It had no effect. I would catch him in my rear view mirror following me at all hours of the day and night.

Speculating that the best plan at this point would be to tell him that I had gotten back with John, my old boyfriend, that I was out of his reach all together, I gave him the sad news. Unfortunately, Mike somehow got ahold of John's phone number. He left death threats on his answering machine. John and I were still friends after a normal break-up. He phoned me laughing hysterically. "What in G-d's name is going on? What's with that guy?"

"I didn't know what else to do so I told him we had gotten back together."

"Well thanks a lot. He's a nut."

"Sorry!" I said.

Mike and I had had a pretty generic relationship. Nothing, not a single red flag had been raised alerting me that he would react in this way. He was intelligent, and pretty laid back throughout our courtship. The chemistry just wasn't there. It was a one-way road as far as love goes. I figured the breakup would only get more difficult as time went on, so why continue?

I always thought, when things go awry in this manner, that there would have been signs of controlling behavior or even violence in the relationship. There had been nothing, as things progressed from bad to worse.

One of our fellow candidates had a graduation party for our class. I pulled up in front of Denise's house. Once inside, music blared, it was wall-to-wall people. The beer flowed freely. It was a good time until Mike arrived. She had a split-level home. I was standing by a set of four stairs that went down into the living room. As he walked by, Mike shoved me, sending me tripping down the stairs. Time to make my exit. I went out to my car and found the back window had been smashed out.

The next morning I called my insurance company. I could get the window fixed, no problem, but this was getting out of hand. I called his sister again, urging her to ask him to leave me alone.

The next day, my tires were slashed. Looking for direction, I called his best friend, Greg, who was also in our class at the Academy. I told him everything that had happened. Quite nonchalantly he added, "when he slashed your tires with a knife, he was trying to find you, but saw your car first." As if this were a perfectly normal event.

In 1983, the word stalker had not yet been conceived. Things like this weren't a media event back then and no one really talked about it. I had however, been keeping a log of all the bizarre occurrences and venting about him to my sister and brother-in-law, Johnny, who was a semi-pro football player.

"Do you want me to talk to him?" Johnny repeatedly asked me.

"No, it's fine, I can handle it." After the tire incident, I gave in, as I was out of ideas.

"Ok, go talk to him." I said. I gave Johnny the address of Mike's apartment.

It was 0800 hours the next morning at the Fire Academy. I took my usual seat in the classroom. In walked Mike—his face was destroyed! Two black eyes, a laceration to his nose, swollen lips, multiple contusions. No part of his face was left unscathed. Holy shit! I thought. On our first break I got Johnny on the phone.

"What the heck happened? You said you were just going to talk to him, his face is destroyed!"

"I talked to him, like you asked."

"You did a lot more than talking." This is the story I finally got out of him.

Mike had met Johnny once, so he brought his brother Jimmie with him when he went to Mike's apartment, as he wanted to make sure Mike would open his door. They walked up the two flights of stairs to his apartment. Johnny waited around the corner in the hallway, as Jimmie knocked on the door.

"Who is it?" Mike asked.

"Democratic Committeeman." Mike opened the door. Jimmie dragged him out into the hallway and Johnny took a few shots to his face and then sent him plummeting down several flights of stairs.

Later that day, Mike had Johnny arrested for battery. He didn't have to stay in jail, but needed to appear in court in front of a judge the next week. I went with him to court.

I explained to the judge the series of events that had occurred and had brought my log book with me. It documented the days and times of everything that had happened, beginning with the hang-up phone calls, the conversations with his sister, to him slashing my tires, etc.

"Why didn't you call the police?" The judge asked.

"I felt like the police had more important things to do, and I tried every avenue to handle it on my own."

"Case dismissed," he said. I truly felt the judge thought Mike deserved everything he got, even though Johnny had confessed to beating him up.

Perhaps I'm an idiot, but I felt sorry for Mike. There he was, standing in a court of law, his face a patchwork of yellow, green and purple bruises, having admittedly been battered by the defendant, who was found innocent due to Mike being a complete ass.

Whenever there is a conflict in our family, no matter how trivial, someone always has the solution—maybe they need a visit from the Democratic Committeemen.